Hypnotherapy
in healthcare

Hypnotherapy in healthcare

by
Jean Murton, Morton Healey
and Matthew Morrissey

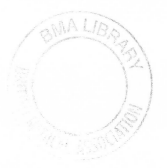

APS Publishing, Fivepin Limited, 91 Crane Street, Salisbury, Wiltshire, UK, SP1 2PU

British Library Cataloguing in Publication Data
A catalogue record for this book is available from the British Library.

© Fivepin Limited 2005
ISBN 1 9038770 5 9

Printed in the United Kingdom by Lightning Source, Milton Keynes

Contents

Introduction

The benefits of hypnotherapy are now being realised and widely used in the healthcare field: hypnotically suggested analgesia (Van Wormer, 2001), hypnosis skills in nursing practice (Kai Tiaki, 2002), use of hypnotherapy with cardiovascular patients (Kreitzer and Snyder, 2002), and specifically in mental health nursing (Zahourek, 2002).

In the UK, it is estimated that one in four of the population will experience a mental health problem at some stage during their life (Klerman, 1987). However, it may be much more prevalent than the figures suggest given that many individuals with acute mental health problems are unlikely to attend a GP or engage a health professional without assistance. Many suffer further the stigma of being mentally ill. Suicide is one of the top ten causes of death in the UK. Defining health or mental health is far from straightforward and it seems the more they are defined, the more elusive their everyday meaning becomes.

The World Health Report (WHO, 2000) defines the objective of good health as two-fold: 'the best attainable average level-goodness and the smallest feasible difference among individuals and groups'. However, this definition has not gone without criticism and some authors claim it is full of paradoxes when you look at health as a global phenomenon (Fernando, 2002). It is not clear what is meant by mental health in a world context. What is clear is that the concept of mental health is much different when considered cross-culturally (White, 1982; Fernando, 2002).

For the purposes of this book it is necessary to provide some working definitions of mental health, mental disorder and types of mental disorder and to outline some common treatments. Unlike many other forms of therapy, the bond between the therapist and client is formed in the initial consultation and all fears and concerns need to be ironed out at this stage for it to work effectively. Many individuals are happily surprised at how relaxed they feel in their first visit. Each individual who has gained insights, hope, and strength through hypnotherapy has their own individual story to reveal: from fear and scepticism at the start, which is normal when trying any new therapy, to the euphoria of an issue resolved.

Some individuals cry in their first session just because they have finally found a support—a person to help them with a specific problem. This is an emotional experience and is often the time when they realise the enormous psychological and emotional burden they have been carrying alone. Although it is a truism that we all need someone to listen to us, the reality is that nurses, doctors and other health professionals often have too little time to spare.

It is time to harness support like hypnotherapy in working closely with people with mental and emotional health needs. It is vital finally to realise the enormous and real potential for hope that hypnotherapy can generate for users. It may be that hypnotherapy will become just one of the therapies being provided by a trust, hospital, or community service in a purpose-built unit. It is clear that already there is a crisis in acute care and a great absence of any real face-to-face therapy (Sainsbury, 1998; 2002).

In reality, it is now clear that some of the major health problems of today are concerned with not just mental, but also emotional health. Many people with mental health problems, including elderly people, have diminished or no real social support networks and may often be lonely and socially disadvantaged (Blacker and Clare, 1987). Many of these people are desperate for skilled help and social contact. Of more concern is the growing trend to find more and more people with serious mental health problems ending up in prison or on the street. More than anything these individuals need resources, hope and practical support.

Historically many voluntary organisations are very much involved with mental health issues. Carers' and users' expectations of services has been the focus of recent psychiatric research (Lelliott *et al*, 2001). However, it is equality that is at the core for users and the need for the creation of an enabling culture which will promote human rights, such as the right to work, the right to speak, the right to have pride in oneself, the right to humane and effective treatment, that is so important. Part of this ought to be to receive therapy that gives them power over their lives—a real choice. Comfort and protection of a person's dignity are important. Nurses can and do benefit from hypnotherapy given their workload and emotional and psychological stress.

Therapy

Mental health should not be just about medication management; it needs to be about forging alliances that will help a user to live, to promote and to create social networks, to have treatment choices, to live a fulfilling life and to have fun. Hypnotherapy can be an important part of new developments for people living with a mental health problem. Our work as therapists can also be about facilitating self-help groups (Bower *et al*, 2001) learning and teaching coping skills, social skills (French, 1983), work skills, relationship skills and survival skills. Hypnotherapists are trained in communication skills, interpersonal skills and crafting trust with individuals. In the time we now live in, it is not unusual for a family to be touched or affected by some serious mental health or emotional problem. The diversity of care requirements is enormous in mental health services. Students of hypnotherapy are being given more and more input on mental health topics to help prepare them for their practice with this client group.

Students of hypnotherapy

Research at the Belmont Centre of Ramsgate, Kent, a centre that specialises in training would-be hypnotherapists and is internationally recognised, suggests that students training as hypnotherapists regard the input of professionals working with people in the mental health field essential to hypnotherapists in training, to identify key boundaries, selection of clients for hypnotherapy, and deal with difficult issues. Questions varied in group discussions but centred around selection, dealing with such complex problems as bi-polar disorders, multiple personality disorders and phobias.

Matthew Morrissey MSc., BSc.(Hons), RMN Dip. Health Ed. MBAThH

Treatments

The main treatments for mental disorder fall into a number of categories: medication, psychological interventions, including psychotherapy, hypnotherapy, counselling, cognitive-behavioural therapy, and nursing interventions. The main types of care for depression, for example, are initially after an assessment, which usually includes a period of observation, then a diagnosis. If the depression is defined as a reactive depression then it needs to be decided if it is best treated psychologically, for example using counselling or some other method. The rates of mental health problems vary, but some researchers have offered a guide (Strathedee *et al*, 1997). However, many students need to read around the subject. References which may be of interest are included in the bibliography (Gamble and Brennan, 2001; Nolen Hoeksema, 2001; Regel and Roberts, 2002; Stuart and Sundeen, 1997; Watkins, 2001).

Mental health disorders

Diagnosis	Rates per 1000 population per year	No of patients per year in a practice of 1900
Schizophrenia	2–6	4–12
Active psychosis	3.0	6–7
Organic dementia	2.2	4–5
Depression	30–50	60–100
Anxiety and other neuroses	35.7	70–80

Diagnosis	Rates per 1000 population per year	No of patients per year in a practice of 1900
Situational disturbances/other diagnoses	26.7	50–60
Drug and alcohol dependency	2.7	5–6
Personality disorder	1.1	2–3

(Strathedee *et al*, 1997)

12

Hypnotherapy in healthcare

A little way in a very long time

In 1843 or thereabouts, Dr John Elliotson, one of the founders of University College Hospital in London, a well-known and highly respected medical doctor, the editor and publisher of the medical journal *The Zoist* and lecturer at London's leading school of medicine, was invited to present the 'Harveian Ovation'.

Elliotson was delighted and flattered. To deliver the Harveian was very prestigious event. Having heard of the work being done in Calcutta by a Dr Esdaile, who was at this time using mesmerism (this was before Dr Braid re-christened it hypnosis) to induce a trance state during which he performed 300 hundred surgical operations, Elliotson decided to base his lecture on the subject of mesmerism. In those days anaesthesia was unknown. Over all the operations that were performed under mesmerism-induced anaesthesia, the mortality rate fell to around 5 per cent instead of the more usual 50 per cent and the patients experienced no pain.

Extreme hostility in past

In those days, within the British medical profession in general, there was extreme hostility towards mesmerism. As a result of his choice of subject for the lecture, Elliotson was ordered to stop using mesmerism in his own hospital. He resigned from his University College Hospital, protesting:

> *This Institution was established for the discovery and dissemination of truth. We should be leading the public, not the public*

leading us. All else is secondary. The sole question is whether it is truth or not.'

The hostility was so extreme that when Esdaile wrote to the British Medical Board four years later, reporting his success in the use of 'Mesmerism—as practised by me', the letter was not even acknowledged.

The leading journal of the medical profession, *The Lancet*, announced its own verdict on this pioneering work in the field of human suffering. 'Mesmerism,' it pronounced, 'is too gross a humbug to admit of any further serious notice. We regard its abettors as quacks and impostors. They ought to be hounded out of professional society' (*The Lancet*, ??vol no??: 24–13).

The man being denounced as a quack and an impostor was described by Dr Sidney van Pelt, a past president of the British Society of Medical Hypnotists, as 'one of the most brilliant men in the history of British medicine'.

Franz Anton Mesmer

Mesmer was born on 23 May 1734, near Lake Constance, on what is now the German side. He was well educated and received a medical qualification at the age of 32. His dissertation was on the influence of heavenly bodies on people's health, which he supposed to be by means of 'animal gravity'.

He was 40 years of age before he became interested in the effects of magnets on the body and believed that he had discovered a new system of healing involving 'animal magnetism'. This 'animal magnetism', he thought, was different from physical magnetism in that he believed that he could 'magnetise' people. His reported cure of Maria Theresa Paradies, when he was 43, was only partially successful and the repercussions of this affair made it necessary for him to move from Vienna to Paris. It was, in fact, the first reported example of a secondary benefit that circumvented a successful original issue, for the move to Paris was to be the scene of his greatest fame. There he met ready acceptance from the populace, but an equally strong scepticism from the medical profession, who attributed the effects he produced to the imagination of the patients rather than to his supposed new force.

So many poor people came for treatment that he had to resort to methods which could help many at once. He first designed a magnetic baquet. The baquet was 'an oaken tub specially designed to store and transmit magnetic fluid. The tub, some four or five feet in diameter and one foot in depth, had a lid constructed in two pieces. At the bottom of the tub, arranged in concentric circles, were bottles, some empty and pointing towards the centre, some containing magnetized water and pointing out towards the circumference. There were several layers of such rows. The tub was filled with water to which iron filings and powdered glass were added. Iron rods emerging through holes in the tub's lid were bent at right angles so that the ends of the rods could be placed against the afflicted areas of the patient's body. A number of patients could use the baquet at one time. They were encouraged to augment the magnetic fluid by holding hands, thus creating a circuit' (Crabtree, 1993; pp.13–14).

Mesmer and suggestion

Mesmer was well aware of the power of suggestion, and although he was convinced that a transfer of healing power was taking place in the use of his 'baquet', he was nevertheless aware that an element of suggestion was also significant. His technique was to dress in flowing robes decorated with the signs of the zodiac. He would enter the room in which his 'patients' were standing around the baquet holding the metal rods that enabled them to connect with the healing power emanating from the baquet. Holding aloft his own metal 'wand' he walked around behind his patients, stopping from time to time to tap one of them on the shoulder and announce, 'You may go. You are cured'. The patient, many of whom were women, would often fall to the floor in a faint.

He finally left Paris at the age of 54 and after some years settled back near Lake Constance where he had been born. Here he seems to have led a quiet and contented life, doing a little medicine, playing his glass harmonica, and remaining detached from the outside world until his death on 15 March 1815, at the age of 85. He never changed his views on animal magnetism but did return to the Catholic Church from which he had lapsed for most of his life.

Hypnotherapy in non-medical practice

Hypnotherapy is a procedure whereby subjects are enabled to access their own unacknowledged potentials, in order to bring about behavioural changes that will make it possible for them to achieve their own healing potential. Hypnotic suggestions can bring about a realisation of unused and previously undeveloped abilities, which, with the proper understanding and teaching, can instigate an endogenous healing process. The hypnotherapist, by carefully and gently investigating the client's lifestyle, background and behavioural patterns, belief systems and prejudices, can, in what would appear to be a casual preliminary chat, assess what life experiences and mental abilities are available within the client's persona to assist in the healing process.

Establishing rapport

Probably the most vital phase of this interview is the establishment of a sound rapport. There must be an experience of empathy, understanding and mutual respect between the therapist and the patient. Without this rapport it is more than likely the therapist will not be able to gather the true facts about the patient's problem due to inhibiting factors relating to the nature of the problem.

It is accepted today that almost 80 per cent of the complaints presented at the GP's surgery are psychosomatic in origin. A large percentage of these are the result of life experiences, largely during childhood. The therapist needs to examine the patient's personal history in order to isolate the sources, or possible sources, of the problem or problems. During this process the therapist is continually asking him or herself, 'What are the filters through which this patient is viewing his/her world?'

Behavioural change

A vital component in the establishment of behavioural change is, without doubt, the creation of an atmosphere of expectancy on the part of both the therapist and the patient. It is interesting to observe the gradual increase of confidence and expectancy, as the patient slowly realises the significance of the early life experiences which are being revealed during an apparently casual chat ranging from early childhood to present day. This increase in expectancy is a most powerful asset of the therapist and is instrumental in enhancing suggestibility to such an extent that the induction of a trance state is greatly facilitated. Almost miraculous-seeming cures are not uncommon.

A waking suggestion

Michael needed to overcome his lack of self-confidence. A tall, slim, dark-haired man of about 30 years with a slight stoop—a civil servant—his sharp features had that tight look which always reveals a high level of inner tension. In our preliminary chat he told me that he was very sceptical about the effectiveness of hypnotherapy but, having 'investigated all avenues of conventional medicine' (his words), he came to hypnotherapy as a last resort.

In order to relieve his anxiety I explained to him the technique I proposed to use in his case and then added, 'This technique is so effective that I could use it to anaesthetise your jaw to the extent that you could go from here to your dentist and have a tooth extracted without anaesthetic and without you feeling a thing'.

As I said this I ran my finger along the side of his jaw. This seemed to calm his anxiety to some extent. I spoke to him for perhaps fifteen minutes more, explaining how and why hypnotherapy worked—something I do with all my clients on their first visit—and then, with his agreement, proceeded with an induction and therapy. He responded well to the induction and I anticipated a successful outcome. When I brought him out of hypnosis and asked him how he felt he opened his mouth and tried without success to speak clearly; he pointed to his jaw and mumbled with difficulty, 'Can't feel a thing'.

At no time during the induction or during the therapy had I said one word about anaesthesia, dentists, or his jaw. His level of expectancy was such that he had accepted the suggestion even when in a state of full consciousness. Of course, this level of suggestibility is not common. An unusual case.

Victor

Victor, an accountant in his own successful business, went to a dinner party with his wife, He was introduced by his host to two of their friends who were hypnotherapists. Unknown to the friends, Victor was due to go into hospital to have an operation on a duodenal ulcer, with which he had suffered for over ten years. It had reached the point where he was unable to eat curries or any kind of rich spicy food. Instead, he ate all kinds of sloppy food because of the pain this ulcer gave him.

As Victor was sitting down, one of the guests, a young woman to whom he had been introduced, asked Victor and his wife if they would mind if she, the guest, might place her hands on Victor's stomach? She had intuitively felt that he was not well, and something was wrong with his stomach. They looked surprised and said, laughingly, 'No, go ahead'.

The young guest then simply placed her hands on to Victor's stomach and suggested that he closed his eyes for a moment and allowed the discomfort to melt away. Everybody carried on talking but he just closed his eyes for a moment. As she placed her hands on to his stomach she was not aware that their hostess was serving curry. After five minutes chatting, the meal was served. Victor sat and ate the curry. He thoroughly enjoyed the meal and everybody was happy, laughing, and joking.

It was not until ten years later that Victor got in touch with Jean who had placed her hands on his stomach. He then told her that he had had an ulcer and, at the time of the party, had an appointment to go into hospital three weeks later, but no one at the dinner party had known about that. The reason he had come to see Jean was to tell her that he had not had to have the operation. Since the party he had had no reoccurrence of the ulcer. He felt he received some form of healing, and mentioned the warmth flowing from the woman's hands. As he imagined the discomfort melting away, he had felt very relaxed. It was the relaxing and the hypnotic suggestion, when he closed his eyes, that he had felt from the warmth and the comfortable feeling of Jean's hands, and when he listened to her suggestions of comfort and well-being, which took away the stress and anxiety: he completely forgot the worry about having to have an operation. The last thing Jean said at that time was, 'Enjoy your meal now. Happy eating'. He could not believe what had happened at that time. He said he had felt guilty not letting Jean know of the healing. Only recently had he become aware that Jean was a very good hypnotherapist. His reason for getting in touch was to ask for her help for a friend with cancer.

Ancient history

Because hypnotherapy has only entered the public domain comparatively recently, it is thought by the majority of the general public to be a new thing. Hypnosis as a medium for healing is one of the oldest of all healing processes. In all the ancient cultures over the past three thousand years, perhaps even longer, techniques of inducing trance states have been used in order to effect cures in cases of serious illness.

Sorcerers, witch-doctors, medicine-men, shamans, voodoo priests and priestesses all practised techniques of trance induction to effect their cures and, by doing so, greatly increased their status and their power over their people.

Hypnosis in Egypt BC

George Ebers, a German Egyptologist, acquired in 1873 a papyrus—the Ebers Papyrus—believed to date from 1550 BC, which described in detail seven hundred treatments used by the high priests of ancient Egypt, including methods of inducing trance states. This papyrus showed a knowledge of the relationship between the heart and the pulse and the circulation of the blood and is believed to be one of the oldest known medical texts.

Even today hypnosis has difficulty in living down its antecedents. For thousands of years its practitioners were workers in the occult and ever since hypnotists have been tarred with the same brush. But in modern times hypnosis is slowly emerging from the shadows. Since the days of Anton Mesmer—who has not spoken of being mesmerised?—the word has become part of our language.

Suggestion all-powerful

Following the work of an English doctor, Richard Mead, Mesmer gave a dissertation in 1766, when he theorised that the gravitational influence of the planetary motions disturbed those fluids within the body which maintained a healthy balance, thus causing dis-ease. He later decided that these influences were 'animal magnetism' rather than gravitation. During the next hundred years many names occur again and again: James Braid (1795–1860), James Esdaile (1808–1859), Elliotson (1791–1868), Coue (1857–1926), all of whom we will meet later in the book. In 1882 two doctors, natives of Troves, France, established a school of hypnosis in the town of Nancy. A student at that school was a pharmacist called Coue who was to become an influential figure in the study of the power of suggestion. He formulated the three rules of suggestion.

1. When logic and emotion are in accord it will not be as though they are added together, but rather as if they are multiplied by each other;

2.   If logic and emotion are not in accord then emotion will always defeat logic; and

3.   Emotions can be changed.

Suggestion is the bedrock of hypnotherapy. Many members of the medical profession deny the capacity of hypnotherapy in the healing process and yet believe implicitly in the placebo effect. If that isn't suggestion, what is it?

The doctor hands the patient a prescription and says, in effect, 'Take the tablet (or whatever) four times a day for seven days.' If the problem is emotionally-based and if the patient likes the doctor and has faith in his ability, there is a 60 per cent chance of recovery, even if the drug in question is not fully effective. The suggestion that has been accepted, although it was not actually spoken, was: 'If you take this medicine for seven days it will cure you'.

In large numbers of double-blind tests run by drug companies, 60 per cent has been the percentage of test subjects, recipients of placebos, who show improvement. In a 1955 study by an anaesthesiologist, Henry Knowles Beecher, involving more than a thousand patients, the condition of 35 per cent of those treated with nothing more than placebos showed improvement. The effectiveness of the placebo effect was not associated with any particular personality types or other psychological characteristics.

Hypnotic anaesthesia

Hypnotherapy has been used successfully in the treatment of pain in many different situations. Victims of severe burns have achieved relief using hypnotic techniques when drugs have proved of no avail. Patients who refuse to accept injections have undergone extremely painful dental procedures while in hypnotic trance states—often self-induced—and felt no pain. The intractable pain of terminal cancer has been relieved using post-hypnotic suggestion.

'From the moment that you hear me clap my hands you will experience a wonderful feeling of comfort and ease. From that moment on you don't feel a thing.'

A medical doctor, Dr Esdaile (1805–1859), practiced in India during the first half of the nineteenth century. He was frequently faced with conditions which demanded surgery, particularly amputations. Anaesthetics were, in those days, unknown. More than half the victims died. Having studied hypnosis he was convinced that it could be used to achieve pain-free surgery. Having perfected his technique, he was able to perform more than three hundred surgical procedures with the patients totally free from pain.

Fatality rate down to five per cent

The fatality rate fell from more than 50 per cent to less than 5 per cent. Esdaile wrote to the British Medical Council (BMC) reporting his results. His letter was not even acknowledged. Some time later, while on leave in England, he offered to demonstrate before a selected audience, the audience to be selected by the BMC, and also a patient regarded by the BMC as suitable. The patient selected was in need of an amputation of the leg above the knee. In those days such operations were performed at great speed in order to get the job done before the patient died. An experienced surgeon could complete the process in three minutes. Esdaile hypnotised his patient and performed the operation without haste and without the patient showing any signs of discomfort. The audience of prominent doctors and surgeons went into a prolonged huddle and finally announced their verdict, 'The patient had fraudulently pretended to feel no pain.'

The 'State' theorists

In spite of huge amounts of various types of evidence, it has proved extremely difficult to convince the medical and the psychological professional bodies that hypnosis is a unique condition, or state of consciousness. Until very recently there existed two bodies of theorists: the 'state' theorists and the 'non-state theorists'.

The most prominent 'state' theory is that of Ernest Hilgard's Neo-dissociation theory (1974; 1977). According to this theory there exist many states of consciousness which do not all function at the same time, but they are regulated by a control function, which ensures that they all maintain a dynamic balance, thus enabling the system to function effectively. In hypnosis, Hilgard maintains that the control function is repressed and the subject's reality is distorted. This condition renders the subject susceptible to suggestion. He refers to this 'control' as the 'hidden observer'.

Hilgard established the Hypnosis Laboratory at Stanford University in 1957. 'By establishing standards for evaluating hypnotic procedures and for measuring hypnotic analgesia, Hilgard and his co-workers demonstrated hypnotic phenomena could be scientifically investigated' (Joseph Barber, 1996).

The 'Non-State' theorists

Those doctors and surgeons who witnessed Esdaile's demonstration were good examples of the 'non-state' view. They believe that the subjects are role-playing; they are acting as they think they are expected to act.

Using all the measuring techniques available to the modern laboratory, it is not difficult to demonstrate that in the hypnotic state physiological changes do occur, but it can be argued that the same changes occur during concentrated attention or in relaxation. There are many hypnotic phenomena which are not possible of this explanation.

In recent times, the 'wind of change' has been blowing very strongly in favour of hypnotherapy in healthcare. Nevertheless, the medical profession in general is still reluctant to give hypnotherapy the credit that it is due. There is a preference to use the term 'placebo effect' to describe the almost miraculous benefits that can be experienced by patients who have accepted suggestions on a conscious level. The suggestion is strengthened by the environment (the doctor's surgery) the white coat, and the stethoscope.

Placebo or suggestion?

Medical doctors sometimes give placebos to patients. Those who believe in the placebo-effect point to clinical research projects in which placebos are used as a control group. It is frequently found that in as much as 60/80 per cent of cases the placebo is as effective as the drug (Kirsch, 1998). Some believe that the effect is due to the patient's belief in the effectiveness of the drug. Irving Kirsch believes that the effectiveness of Prozac® and similar drugs may be almost 100 per cent due to the placebo effect. In trials analysed by Guy Sapirstein and Kirsch between 1974 and 1995, of 39 cases of depressed patients treated with drugs, psychotherapy or both, Sapirstein found that 50 per cent of the drug effect is due to the placebo effect.

A patient's belief and their faith in the treatment, reinforced by their suggestibility, may have a profound biochemical effect. The body's hormonal and immune systems are affected by the patient's belief and may be very important to their physical well-being and recovery from illness. If one considers that a person's susceptibility to suggestion is greatly increased when in hypnosis, it would be reasonable to accept that a skilful hypnotherapist would be able to offer such suggestions to the patient's subconscious, thus enabling the placebo effect to be many times more powerful.

'Warts and All'

In an article *The Placebo Prescription* by Margaret Talbot in the *New York Times Magazine*, 9 January 2000, she reported:

> *'Doctors in one study successfully eliminated warts by painting them with a brightly coloured inert dye and promising the patients the warts would be gone when the colour wore off. In a study of asthmatics, researchers found that they could produce dilation of*

the airways by simply telling people they were inhaling a bronchiodilator even when they weren't. Patients suffering pain after wisdom tooth extraction got just as much relief from a fake application of ultrasound as from a real one, so long as both patient and therapist thought the machine was on; 52 per cent of colitis patients treated with placebos in 11 different trials reported feeling better—and 50 per cent of the inflamed intestines actually looked better when assessed with a sigmoidoscope.'

All these effects are achieved with the patient in a state of full consciousness. How much more effective would they be if the suggestion was given directly to the subconscious? The suggestion then works subliminally.

Subliminal suggestion—fact or fiction

Examples of the way in which we use subliminal suggestion in conjunction with a post-hypnotic suggestion will be found in Chapter 6: 'From the moment that I tell you to wake up again today you feel no need, no desire, no craving for cigarettes or tobacco in any form.' When your client is in hypnosis that suggestion goes directly into the client's subconscious mind. For all our therapies we always give a minimum of two sessions— how can you know that the first session has been successful if you do not see them again? On attending for the second session people frequently comment on the fact that they did not even realise that they had not smoked for several hours. The effect had been subliminal. This is not only true of smokers but of almost all our treatments: eating disorders, anxiety states, alcoholism, confidence, and all the many psychosomatic disorders we meet from day to day. But, of course, the use of subliminal suggestion in this context is very different from subliminal *advertising* which has been the subject of such a long debate.

In 1957 Vance Packard published a book, *The Hidden Persuaders*. It was the general public's first introduction to subliminal advertising. He did not describe it as subliminal advertising, but he did describe many of the new marketing techniques being employed by advertising agents to sell products in the post-war American market—advertisements that contained hidden messages which targeted consumers' hopes, fears, guilt, and sexuality and were designed to persuade them to buy products they'd never initially intended to buy.

It was James Vicary who coined the term 'subliminal advertising'. Vicary had conducted a variety of unusual studies of female shopping habits. None are worthy of note for our purposes except for the experiment he conducted at a New Jersey movie theatre during the summer of 1957. He placed a tachistoscope in the theatre's projection booth, and all throughout the playing of the film *Picnic*, he flashed two different messages on the screen every five seconds. The messages were each displayed for only a fraction of a second at a time, far below the viewers' threshold of conscious perception. The result of displaying these subliminal suggestions— 'Drink Coca-Cola' and 'Hungry? Eat Popcorn'—was reported to be an amazing 18.1 per cent increase in Coca-Cola sales, and a huge 57.8 per cent jump in popcorn sales; thereby demonstrating the power of 'subliminal advertising' to persuade buyers into making purchases they would not otherwise have made.

A second experiment

Therein started the debate that has continued for almost 50 years. The then president of the Psychological Corporation, Dr Henry Link, challenged Vicary to repeat his experiment but Vicary was unable to demonstrate any significant increase in sales of either Coca Cola or of popcorn when responding to this challenge. It is reported that Vicary lied about the results of his experiment. He is said to have confessed that he had falsified the data from his first experiment. There is, however, some doubt about this report. In 1974 the Federal Communications Commission (FCC) banned 'subliminal advertising' from radio and television despite the fact that no studies have ever shown it to be effective, and even though its efficacy was allegedly based on a fraud. At the time of the first experiment, the media made much of what was a sensational story. Until then no one had ever heard of 'subliminal suggestion', but by the time of the second experiment most of the cinema going public were aware of it. Could the second experiment genuinely be said to be an exact replica of the first? Would there have been subconscious rejection of a subliminal suggestion?

Subliminal seduction

The public memory is notoriously short. In 1958 and 1959 two bills were introduced to Congress with the aim of banning 'subliminal advertising'; neither was even voted upon. But then the sleeping dog was kicked into life. A Doctor Wilson B Key published *Subliminal Seduction*: an indictment of contemporary publishing which he claimed was full of advertisements containing 'hidden messages and secret codes'—messages that only he (Dr Key) had been able to decipher, but which were capable of influencing the buying public without their knowledge.

This led to the announcement in January 1974, by the FCC, that 'subliminal techniques, whether effective or not, were contrary to the public interest, and that any station employing them risked losing its broadcast license.'

Although there is a considerable background of experimental proof to support the existence of subliminal perception, there is a lack of scientific theories of human physiology to support the case. Medical research has only recently begun to investigate the inner functioning of the human brain. Psychologist N F Dixon, (1971) contends that because through millions of years our brain has evolved from unconscious processing—i.e. driven only by survival and procreation—to conscious awareness, the brain has developed control mechanisms to filter most of the sensory input. 'To fully utilize the limited consciousness, and to protect the brain from sensory overload, only a fraction of the sensory input is channeled into the conscious mind. The rest is processed by our unconscious mind.' He writes:

'It is contended that the principles of physiological summation, inhibition, and facilitation, the notion of interactions between specific and non-specific effects, and the existence of centrifugal-centripetal "gating" loops within the central nervous system,

provide all that is necessary for a viable theory, without recourse to any concept that is anthropomorphic or supernatural.'

He argues that there is physiological evidence for the possibility of subliminal perception, but the research is not thorough enough to prove its existence.

As with every theory, there are those who deny the possibility of subliminal perception. Curiously, the loudest voices come from the advertising industry. The most often used argument is that it is inherently unlikely, physiologically inexplicable, and based upon anecdotal evidence. There are many plausible reasons why people vehemently deny the existence of this phenomenon. Could it be that the advertising industry does not want people to believe that subliminal advertising is possible? People instinctively fear what they do not know. We live in a country where personal freedom is one of the founding principles of this democratic society. To admit to subliminal influences is to admit to the fact that there are areas of our brain that we cannot ourselves control, but which can be influenced without our knowledge. That thought can be very frightening. That is why we—the hypnotherapists— must understand about subliminal advertising.

The Achilles Heel

The subliminal techniques advertisers use to influence the buying public are focused on the vulnerabilities of the human minds they target. We are all vulnerable in some way. Even the greatest of all Greek warriors, Achilles, who was said to be impregnable because his mother, Thetis, had dipped him in the river Styx when he was a baby, had his vulnerable spot. Thetis held him by his heel as she dipped him in the Styx. Only by a wound on his heel could he be killed. In the Trojan war an arrow shot by Paris pierced his heel and Achilles died. We all have our Achilles Heel. As hypnotherapists it is our job to understand those issues and help people to overcome them.

Advertisers use subliminal techniques to target the consumer's fears and desires, manipulating them in ways never before thought possible. But to the casual observer or reader, the consumer is, on a conscious level, viewing or reading a normal persuasive advertisement; it rarely receives close scrutiny, it has been seen so many times before. These are the optimum conditions for subliminal reception because the conscious mind is not really concentrating—critical judgement is suspended.

To know the difference

The greatest obstacle to success in the use of hypnotherapy is the client/patient's fear of hypnosis—the fear of losing control of their own minds; fear of being made to do or say something that they would not do or say in a state of full consciousness. The general public have many misconceptions about hypnotherapy and the massive publicity given to subliminal advertising emphasised this anxiety. The knowledge that subliminal advertising had been made illegal confirmed in the public's mind that this was a dangerous practice and few people had the knowledge to differentiate between subliminal advertising and *subliminal response*.

This situation is compounded by the fact that a very large percentage of the problems presented to the hypnotherapist are founded in fear. It is our job to enable people to conquer their fears.

2

The healing power of hypnosis

It could almost be called common knowledge, today, that hypnotherapy can very effectively help people to stop smoking, to lose weight, to overcome anxiety states, or to cure nail biting, but not so well known is that there are far greater benefits to be gained by using hypnotherapy in the treatment of serious health problems.

For a very long time forms of hypnosis have been used in the treatment of serious illness, as illustrated in the Ebers Papyrus, for example discovered by George Ebers (*Chapter 1*, p.4). In spite of this there has been a strange dearth of information on the subject in the medical literature of the past two or three hundred years. The difficulty we face is the same for the medical profession as for the great mass of the public at large.

What is mind?

Hypnosis is aimed at relaxing the unconscious, which some say controls the mind. Anxiety is a state of the mind, and habits such as nail biting, and even smoking are influenced by the strength of will that exists in our minds. But what has mind got to do with really serious disorders like cancer or MS, or a bacterial or viral infection? After all, some very important people in the world of science don't believe that such a thing as mind really exists; they believe only in the brain. Mind is an abstract concept. It cannot be seen or touched; it does not occupy any space. We talk glibly of 'mind over matter' without believing that what we call mind really could affect matter. We accept that high levels of stress will have deleterious affects upon our immune system. We know that people with stomach ulcers, eczema, asthma, and heart disease suffer increased discomfort when experiencing stress. It is not difficult for Mr General Public to accept that hypnosis, by inducing deep levels of relaxation, can alleviate the symptoms of these ailments, but what about a disease such as cancer? Is it possible that the power of the mind reinforced by hypnosis could defeat cancer? Some doctors believe so.

Victory for the subconscious

Dr Cangello does. In the 1962 *American Journal of Clinical Hypnosis* 4: 215–26, Cangello presented a case of leukaemia:

> *A fifty year old female, with leukaemia had had many hospital admissions of considerable length and was seen three weeks after a splenectomy, which had produced a dramatic remission of her disease. She had a very stormy postoperative course, complicated by wound infection. She was severely depressed and anorexic. A hypnotic induction was done using disguised technique. Suggestion of good appetite and well-being were given. There was dramatic improvement in her mental state and her appetite improved. She was discharged within two weeks. She was seen six months later and stated she had experienced peculiar food desires for three months after her discharge from hospital. At this time the patient was still enjoying a remission from her disease and looked and felt extremely well.*

But Cangello was by no means a first. In 1848, Dr Elliotson (see *Chapter 1*) reported a case study of his treatment of a case of advanced breast cancer in the medical journal, *The Zoist*. The article was entitled, 'A cure of a true cancer of the female breast with Mesmerism'. Mesmerism was of course the precursor of hypnotism and was only known as hypnotism after it was so christened by Dr Braid (circa 1855). Elliotson reported:

> *In March 1843 a woman of middle age, a Miss Barber, complained of a disease of her right breast. I found a very hard tumour in her breast; it was movable and about two inches in diameter. The area was drawn in and puckered and on the outer*

19

side of the nipple was a dry rough warty looking matter, dirty brown and greenish in appearance. She complained that it was extremely tender in the tumour and in the armpit when palpated and said she had sharp stabbing pains through the tumour during the day and was continually awakened by them during the night. I saw at once that it was a decided cancer in the stage named Cirrhus. I did not explain the nature of the tumour to her. On enquiry I found that in November 1841 having raised her right hand she felt a sudden sharp violent pain in her right breast. A week later she experienced it again. These dreadful darting pains began to happen a dozen times in rapid succession and every few hours. Her nights were disturbed and pricking sensations and great tenderness always followed the darting pains. Fomenting it with warm water gave some relief but she found that it had become hard. Her complexion and her hands had become sallow. For many months she described it to her doctor but declined to show it to him because he was young. Her father's mother had died of bleeding cancer of the breast. I proposed Mesmerism to her. My purpose was to render her insensible to the pain of the surgery of breast removal seeing no other chance for her, and this was a poor chance, for cancer invariably returns in the same or some other part if the patient survives long enough and the operation is not to be recommended unless it can be conducted without pain. When a condition which has been diagnosed, as cancer does not return I have no doubt that it had been wrongly diagnosed and was not cancer. Such a terrible thing as removal of a breast not cancerous, has always been too frequent among surgeons.

Unwilling to make her unhappy, I said no more and allowed her to suppose that the mesmerism was intended to cure her disease. I mesmerised her for half an hour daily. Her eyes perfectly closed and she fell asleep near the expiation of the half hour. At the end of the month her pain had lessened so that her nights became greatly better and her health and spirits improved.

For the first six months the tumour increased and she could work no more. At her mother's request she showed her breast to her doctor who immediately pronounced it to be a confirmed incurable cancer, adding that if it were not cut away it would be as big as his head by Christmas and that if mesmerism could cure it he would believe anything. Thus she learnt the distressing truth, which I had been anxious to keep from her.

Cure; a bonus

By the end of the summer of 1844, the sallowness vanished. She had much less pain and her general health improved. The external growth around the nipple dropped off leaving clean skin beneath. During the four years of constant treatment it was necessary for Elliotson to make occasional trips abroad. During these absences he arranged for a locum to continue the daily periods of mesmerism. This was not an unqualified success and some regression occurred but when Elliotson resumed treatment the improvement was regained and Miss Barber's condition improved in every respect; the cancerous mass began to reduce. In the summer of 1845 a Dr Engledue saw her and diagnosed the condition as cancer.

A year later the pain was non-existent. The tumour continued to shrink and by the end of 1847, it completely disappeared. The breast became perfectly normal and all associated tenderness was gone. (*Zoist*, 1848).

It is worthy of note that even Elliotson himself did not expect to achieve a complete cure. He was treating Miss Barber in order to achieve some level of anaesthesia when she eventually had to endure surgery. In the event this never became necessary—this at a time when the *Lancet* was describing Mesmerism as '...too gross a humbug to admit of any further serious notice' (*Chapter 1*, p.2).

But notice was being taken. Members of the the British Medical Association of the day were not all dinosaurs and in the British Medical Journal of 29 July 1893, we see the following article:

Report of the Committee Appointed to Investigate the Nature of the Phenomena of Hypnotism; its Value as a Therapeutic Agent; and the Propriety of using it

The Committee, having completed such investigation of hypnotism as time permitted, has to report that they have satisfied themselves of the genuineness of the hypnotic state. No phenomena, which have come under their observation, however, lend support to the theory of 'animal magnetism'.

The experiments, which have been carried out by members of the Committee, have shown that this condition is attended by mental and physical phenomena, and that these differ widely in different cases. Among the mental phenomena are: altered consciousness, temporary limitation of willpower, increased receptivity of suggestion from without, sometimes to the extent of producing passing delusions and hallucinations, an exalted condition of the attention, and post hypnotic suggestions.

Among the physical phenomena are vascular changes (such as flushing of the face and altered pulse rate), deepening of respirations, increased frequency of deglutition, slight muscular tremors, inability to control suggested movements, altered muscular sense, anaesthesia, modified power of muscular contraction, catalepsy, and rigidity, often intense. It must however be understood that all these mental and physical phenomena are rarely present in any one case. The Committee take this opportunity of pointing out that the term 'hypnotism' is somewhat misleading inasmuch as sleep, as ordinarily understood, is not necessarily present.

The Committee are of the opinion that, as a therapeutic agent, hypnotism is frequently effective in relieving pain, procuring sleep, and alleviating many functional ailments. As to its efficacy in the treatment of drunkenness, the evidence before the Committee is encouraging, but not conclusive. Dangers in the use of hypnotism may arise from want of knowledge, carelessness, or intentional abuse, or from the too continuous repetition of suggestions in unsuitable cases.

The Committee are of the opinion that when used for therapeutic purposes its employment should be confined to qualified medical men and that under no circumstances should female patients be hypnotised except in the presence of a relative or a person of their own sex.

In conclusion, the Committee desire to express their strong dis-

approbation of public exhibitions of hypnotic phenomena, and
hope that some legal restriction will be placed upon them.

Signed: F Needham Chairman
T Outerson Wood Hon Sec

A four-year battle

We are not given any detailed information about the techniques of mesmerism used by Elliotson in treating Miss
Barber, but the thought of daily half-hour sessions over a
period of four years seems inconceivable to the author who, if
he has to consider giving a fourth session, is beginning to
think that he is doing something wrong. However, if, as was
the case for Miss Barber, one is faced with the options of:

(a) a hideously painful mastectomy with the very low probability of a successful outcome,

(b) a slow painful death from the breast cancer and the inevitable metastases,

(c) Daily sessions of mesmerism for as long as may be necessary with the probability of relief from pain and the possibility of a complete cure,

...there is little doubt which option one would choose.

More effective techniques

Fortunately we are equipped with more effective and more
efficient techniques than those with which Elliotson had to
operate and with our greater knowledge of how and why
hypnotherapy works, it is possible to achieve successful outcomes in much less time. It is really remarkable that
hypnotherapy was used with such success in those early days.
In his book, *Treatment By Hypnotism And Suggestion*, (1989), Dr
Charles Lloyd Tuckey describes in detail 35 of his own case
histories with 34 successful outcomes. This is a book of 450

pages and on almost every other page can be found one or more cases.

A Swish Technique

If we want to understand the ideodynamic methods of healing and hypnosis, this is written up indepth in *The Mind/Body Therapy that is of the Ideodynamic Healing in Hypnosis* by Ernest L Rossi and David B Cheek. A question was asked, 'Does ideodynamic signalling really reach deeper into our psycho/ biological matrix to access sources of mind/body healing not usually available to verbally-oriented psychotherapy?' Most of us have a fairly naïve conception of the nervous system. It is usually likened to a telephone exchange. A stimulus from the outside world brings a response to a sense organ, which in turn transmits impulses along the nerves to our brain, like messages through a telephone wire. We know that nerves are neurons and are separated from one another by small gaps called synapses, and that neuro-transmitters carry the message across synapses from one neuron to another. This is called neuro-transmission. It has also been discovered in recent times that there are hormonal messenger molecules—also called information substances—that modulate neuro-transmission. These are the neuro-modulators which stimulate or inhibit neuron action, as well as the activity of most other cell tissue and organ systems of the body (Bloom, 1986; Iverson, 1986; Schmitt, 1984). The profound differences between neuro- transmission and neuro-modulation for ideodynamic healing is what we use in hypnosis. Research has also found significant developments in psychobiology, memory learning and behaviour (Gold, 1987; Izquierdo and Dias, 1984; Mcgaugh, 1983; Stuart 1985; Zornetzer, 1978). It has been discovered that hormonal information substances, released by the stress of any new life situation, can act as neuro-modulators. These information substances can modulate the action of neural systems of the brain so as to encode memory and learning in a special manner.

During the shock and stress of a car accident, for example, the special complex of information substances that are suddenly released by the lymphatic, hypothalamic, pituitary, and the adrenal system encodes all external and internal sensory (visionary, auditory, kinesectic, propioceptive, etc) impressions of the accident in a special state of consciousness. The accident victim is often recognised as being dazed and/or in an altered state of psycho-physiological shock. Hypnotherapists describe such a shock as hypnoidal. The memories of these traumatic events are said to be deeply imprinted as physiological memory, tissue memory or muscle memory. We propose that all these designations are actually metaphors for the special state-dependant encoding of memories by the stress released by these hormonal information substances.

When accident victims recover from their acute trauma and return to 'normal' psycho-physiological states a few hours or days later, they find to their surprise that the details of the accident that were so vivid when it took place are now quite vague or forgotten. This is because the special complex of stress-releasing information substances that have encoded their traumatic memories has changed with their body/mind returning to normal; the memories are thus available in normal consciousness. We say they are experiencing a traumatic amnesia. That the traumatic memories are still present and active, however, is evidenced by the fact that they may influence the accident victim's dreams, but may, for example, be expressed as psychosomatic problems. Different responses to these situations depend upon the age of the person and the degree to which they have responded to the traumatic situation and with the level of emotional support in a therapy situation. These situations range from a birth trauma to child abuse, molestation, shell shock, battle conditions, upheavals and deprivation, and it depends on the personality as to how dramatic and traumatised the person will become.

What does the hypnotherapist do to enable the client to resolve these problems? He/she enables the patient to focus their attention on the reliving of the sensory details, emotions and circumstances of these 'special life events' and can, by association, access their recovered memory encoding. When a client is traumatised, the condition which then exists is known as the 'flight, fright and freeze' state. A victim involved in an accident, a sudden attack or a traumatic situation will feel as if time has stood still—everything seems to be happening in slow motion and seems as if it is never going to stop. In reality it only happens in seconds. In the therapy situation, it is possible to enlist a rewind technique. When in a hypnotic trance state, the victim is told to visualise the situation five minutes before the trauma happened. They are instructed to imagine themselves sitting in an empty cinema, watching the screen on which the trauma situation that they have suffered is now developing. They have in their hands a control with three buttons: start, stop, and rewind. They are told to push the start button when they are ready to run the movie through in their minds. They then visualise the action taking place on the screen from the time a few minutes before it happened, right up to the event taking place. Having watched this imagery from start to finish, the rewind button is pressed and they see the whole event in reverse. This whole process is repeated several times until the victim announces it is no longer causing emotional distress.

This is a disassociated technique where you get the client to imagine themselves a couple of minutes before the start of the process that caused the distress, e.g. before the fear of birds or the trauma happened.

Early techniques

Tuckey's teacher and mentor was Dr Ambroise Liebault, who also taught Sir Francis R Cruise MD, and it was in the fifth edition of Tuckey's book (1907) that Sir Francis wrote a foreword in which he describes the induction used by Liebault. In Sir Francis' words:

> *'Let us suppose ourselves in M Liebault's consulting room. From seven in the morning he worked. He was a remarkably bright, intelligent old gentleman. Simple, kindly in manner, and sympathetic with all his patients who streamed in to seek his aid, mostly when all other means of cure had failed.*

*There were there to be seen countless phases of disease, affect-ing men and women of all ages and many children. His proce-dure was as follows: He placed the patients in turn in an easy reclining chair, with their backs to the light, questioned them closely as to their symptoms and sufferings, and then forthwith hypnotized them. His method was to make the subject stare at his two fingers which he placed a few inches from their eyes, and as soon as the eyes began to water and the pupils to dilate he sug-gested "Sleep" in an emphatic manner, and then closed the eyelids by gently pressing the eyeballs. **In nearly every case**, sooner or later, the patient passed into sleep—of very varying degrees, no doubt; but to all he **suggested verbally** that on awakening their symptoms would be improved.'*

Although there was a great deal of interest among a relatively small number of doctors during the late nineteenth century and throughout most of the twentieth century, in general, the medical profession was violently opposed to hypnosis and did not accept it as a viable therapeutic agent. Witness the attitude of the BMA towards Elliotson. But the shortest distance between two points may not always be a straight line.

A secondary benefit

As an example of the pitfalls awaiting the hypnotherapist, con-sider the dynamics of the following alcoholic problem. As a result of childhood sexual abuse, a woman hated sex when she got married. She could only tolerate it if she was drunk. After a while it followed that if she were to stop or even reduce drink-ing, her husband would perceive her as being in a 'worse' state and consciously or unconsciously encourage her to drink again. Drunk she was sexually active, sober she was frigid. The devil and the deep blue sea.

A secondary benefit 2

There was a still harder lesson to learn in the use of suggestion as a healing therapy, and it was Mesmer who was probably the first to learn the lesson that all is not as it seems. He was called upon to treat a blind musician.

This classic example from the annals of hypnosis involved Mesmer's treatment of the young woman, Maria Theresa Paradies, who had been blind from an early age. She was also a gifted pianist and musician. There are various accounts of this case in circulation, but the main features are as follows. Mesmer had some good initial success, but to his amazement, the parents objected very strongly and removed her from treatment. Then:

> *'The logic is that Paradies* [the father] *began to anticipate serious embarrassment if Maria Theresa was saved from blindness. Her music already suffered from the improvement of her eyes. Partial sight made her nervous at the piano; nervousness made her hit the wrong keys, and the deterioration of her playing made her more nervous. It was a vicious circle from which she could not hope to escape except after long, arduous experience—if then. Meanwhile, she would cease to be the accomplished, petted star of the concert stage with a handsome income of her own. She might lose the pension granted by the empress* [her godmother] *in consideration of her blindness. She would then become a half-crippled burden on her parents.'*

Buranelli (1975)

Clearly there were quite a few consequences of an improvement in sight which were unfavourable to Maria Theresa and her family. The natural result was to react against the improvement, and to return to the status quo. In short, a negative feedback loop was revealed.

The outcome of the case was that her parents took her home from Mesmer's house where he had been treating her, and the condition of her eyes promptly deteriorated again. In outline the pattern was the one-sided negative feedback loop'

However, this story has an ending which should be a caution to all therapists. Mesmer was furious that his cure should have been undermined. But what of Maria Theresa? How did her life proceed?

She went back to her concert life and was a great success in Paris and London. She was so good that Mozart wrote a composition especially for her, the Concerto in B Flat Major. In other words the lack of sight did not blight her life, and might indeed have made it in many ways more fulfilling. Music may well have been all the more beautiful as a result of there not being any visual distractions. She would have had servants to do all the boring, practical things in life. She had music and friends and fame. Was life so very bad? We should beware of thinking that the improvement of a particular symptom by our technique must be the best thing for the client.

The Belmont Way

This is an eclectic technique designed by Jean Murton to accommodate those clients who have a strong resistance to relaxation because they fear that they may be in danger of revealing something that is a closely guarded secret. In the Belmont Way, it is possible to assure the client that they will not be asked what the issue is for which they need therapy. This technique is so powerful that many of the students who have qualified through the Belmont Centre find themselves using it as their induction of choice.

> The client is asked to think of a happy memory, and when they have thought of it bring it close to their eyes. The therapist then says: "Now imagine yourself stepping into that image. See what you are seeing, hear what you are hearing smelling any smells touching or tasting, making it as real as if you are right there making it brighter and clearer and imagine yourself there right NOW."
>
> "Lift your finger when you feel you are there. But keep your eyes closed."

(Ideomotor system)

When the client does this, the therapist helps the client by anchoring that moment, pressing the knuckle gentle and suggesting to the client that they are really in that situation.

"Now," (pause) "allow that feeling to flow right through the whole of your body and when you feel you are there, open your eyes and come back."

We can then test that particular memory by touching the knuckle again; if correctly done, the client will immediately feel that lovely wonderful feeling again. This will be repeated twice.

"Now think of a place of nature. Hear the sounds of nature... Any smells of nature...seeing the beauty of nature ... touching , tasting, make it as real as if you are there right NOW."

Clients put themselves in and out of trance, which increases their ability to go deeper if it is necessary. The therapist is only coaching clients into this state. This reassures them that the therapist does not have the magic power of affecting any changes, either therapeutically or otherwise.

This experience leaves clients with a positive reaction to fall back on should any suggestions given to them cause a negative reaction.

Having achieved the first part of the Belmont Way, we move to the second part of the therapy, using the ideomotive system. The therapist will tap the knuckle on the opposite hand.

She now ask the client to bring forth that part of him/herself that is anxious to be present (i.e. smoker, anxious, depressed issue, etc.)

"When you have found this part, lift your finger."

When the client lifts his/her finger the therapist then will anchor the knuckle. At this point the therapist will tap the knuckle each time the client responds to an emotional issue until they reach the core. The therapist asks the client:

"Is this emotion a punishing or a rewarding feeling?"

The client will respond with either of those emotional issues. It does not matter if it is rewarding or punishing. Whichever the client responds to, the therapist will tap the finger on the anchor and continue to ask the client:

"How does that make you feel emotionally?"

The client may respond with an emotional statement; the therapist continues, asking the question:

"And how does that make you feel?"

The therapist continues to tap the finger until he/she can see and hear that the client has reached the core of an emotional state from a childhood memory, or a more recent trauma. The therapist tells the client:

"You didn't learn this emotion now, you learnt this when you were a child. You may not remember exactly when, but the memory will pop up into your mind as you are regressed."

The therapist will then proceed with age regression:

"I want you to create in your imagination a pathway of light, which is translucent and stretching right out in front of you; imagine yourself standing in the middle of the pathway of light, looking at the future as it stretches away in front of you."

The therapist will then ask the client to:

"Turn yourself around in your mind's eye, and imagine yourself looking back, walking along the pathway, looking down at your past."

The therapist will be gently tapping the finger, in time with the heartbeat; as the client continues to go back in time, he/she listens to the therapist's voice, which keeps the client's mind on the issue at hand. The therapist asks the client to lift a finger to indicate when he/she feels he/she has reached a situation from the past where he/she feels that he/she had been unhappy or upset. The therapist then asks:

"What age do you think you are approximately?"

The therapist continues:

> "Now look down through that pathway of light at yourself at the age or time of that child's situation, when you had this emotional experience."

> "Imagine the child's situation, or remember the love that the child needed at that time. Imagine yourself being like a 'God' and giving that child all the love that it needed at that time. Help the child to forgive any judgements it may have made, about the situation, letting go of any injustices that may have been around it at this time. The one thing that is positive is that YOU survived, and can now let go of the significance of the past."

The therapist is waiting for a signal from the client when he/she has completed this time, by lifting his/her finger once.

When the client indicates by lifting the finger that he/she has resolved this issue, the therapist then asks the client to:

> "Bring that good feeling through to any other situations that you feel will heal your body of any emotional issues. When you want me to stop just lift your finger once."

The therapist continues to tap the finger through the years, telling the client that each time he/she wishes to stop, to lift a finger and, when completed, to lift the finger twice, all the time repeating the process of giving love to the child/parent/peer.

When the client indicates he or she has completed and reached the present age, he or she lifts the finger twice.

At this point we thank the part that needed the help and the client then relaxes. The therapist touches the positive finger and asks the client:

> "I want you to create in your mind the kind of person you would like to be. When you have that person, indicate with your finger (ideomotor system) the part that is present."

The therapist will then tap the finger that has been indicated and say to the client:

> "I want you to create three behaviours that will help the 'issue' part to change its habit."

When the client indicates with her finger that she has three behaviours, the therapist then asks her:

"What is the first suggestion you wish to offer to the part that needs to change?"

"I want to be healthy" the client replies.

The therapist offers this suggestion to the part that had the issue and asks that part:

"Will you accept this suggestion?"

The client replies, "Yes."

"Will this fit in with your environment?" the therapist asks.

The three behaviours that the client has created with the positive aspect are offered to the 'issue part'. When all are excepted the completion process of the Belmont Way is next.

As this technique has disassociated the clients from themselves, we need to associate and bring together the new self without the issue. The therapist asks the client again:

"Now imagine yourself in a court room, and the two parts of yourself are looking at the commitment you have made, written on a golden contract. See these two parts of yourself signing the contract."

"Now."

At the moment of saying 'Now', the therapist crashes the right and left hand anchors at the same time, thus enhancing and associating the change the client wanted.

The therapist tells the client:

"See yourself in the future behaving in this new way for the rest of the day."

When the client indicates by lifting their positive anchor, the therapist says again:

"See yourself in one week with these new behaviours."

When the client indicates that he/she has done so,

"Now in a month."

The client indicates in the same way, each time the client indicates the therapist is anchoring and reinforcing the change by future pacing.

"Now in a year."

At this point and on the count of five, the therapist will bring the client back from the trance state he/she has achieved, reinforcing with positive affirmations.

Hypnotherapy has helped the client to discover his/her own power and recover a resource from his/her own mind, an imprint of his/her positive imagery. The mind has accepted the suggestion, and this brings about the changes.

An agoraphobic

This is a case study where using a simplistic technique has changed a client's belief system.

> Pam, a woman in her 60s, was brought to the clinic by her daughter. She had suffered for over four years with terrible headaches; she had not been able to sleep at night, could not eat, suffered with vertigo, and was agoraphobic. She had reached a point where she was unable to do anything for herself.
>
> Pam had been to specialists, doctors, psychologists, and psychiatrists. She had seen every doctor who could possibly see her and not one of them had been able to help free her of her headaches. Her daughter had heard of a hypnotherapist down the road and thought this was a last chance. They had tried everything else. I was aware of the state of the client as Pam entered the room. She looked very stressed and terrified. I directed Pam to a comfortable chair. She flopped into the chair and sat looking very strained and uncertain. Her face was flushed and she was perspiring as she raised her hands up to her head, and wiped her forehead with a tissue. I then said to her in a caring voice:
>
> "Would you like me to get rid of that headache?"
>
> Pam's startled outcry was, "Yes, yes please."

I then used a simple hypnosis technique.

"Now close your eyes, and go into the centre of the discomfort. Nod your head when you have done that."

Pam nodded her head.

"Now move that discomfort to the right or left, but keep in the centre."

Pam nodded her head. once more.

"Now move it back the other way but keep in the centre."

She nodded her head again.

"Now move that discomfort up underneath the scalp nearest to where the area is and stay in the centre"

Pam was looking less strained in following the instructions, which she did again.

"Now feel that discomfort half an inch to an inch outside the scalp, but keep in the centre."

Again Pam followed the instructions.

"Now feel the discomfort moving away and keep in the centre."

Pam opened her eyes, startled, scared: "Oh my God it's gone. How did you do that? Will it come back? Don't let it come back."

Pam was relieved for the first time in four years. She was panic-stricken that it was going to come back, but what I had done had taken away the headache, a very simple headache. Removing the headache had eliminated the fear from the client and then the story unfolded.

If the medical doctors had taken the time to question Pam, they would have discovered that she was suffering from a psychosomatic disorder. On talking to her she disclosed this feeling of guilt.

I asked her to imagine that if this feeling had a shape, what shape would she give it? If it had a colour what colour? If it had a sound what would it sound like? If it had a smell what would it smell like? Using this kind of metaphor eliminates the actual situation of the feelings. The next suggestion is using whatever faith or belief a client may have. Pam had a belief in God. I used the analogy of the sun being very important to the earth and what would happen if the sun didn't shine—nothing on the earth can live without the sunshine.

"Imagine now that the sun is shining down upon you like a beam of pure light, feel it flowing through you and dissolving away the shape and changing the colour, smell, sound to become small, and then see it melt completely away, leaving you feeling good."

Pam looked so relax, and was beaming when she opened her eyes. The feeling of relief was obvious.

On the second visit, Pam admitted that she had begun to hate her husband and had been on the point of not doing any more for him. Pam was a very independent person, and feeling the way she had for the past four years, it seemed like a miracle that the headache had gone. She had worked hard all her life. She was talented and able to deal with problems. She would do anything for anybody, the WI, the Round-table, Rotary Clubs and she would bend over backwards to help anybody and everybody.

She had been married for 40 years to a man she adored and had two children and everything was wonderful. Her husband had been in the Army and when he came out of the Army he had to find a job. She carried on working harder, enjoying doing what she always did. Her husband got a job with a large company. It was not too bad but it was shift work and he began to get tired and upset; then he discovered that he had diabetes. Pam carried on looking after him, sorting out his diet and doing everything for him. After five years he had a stroke and this paralysed him. Gradually he improved and Pam carried on caring for him. He was left paralysed down one side of his body, which meant he was unable to walk and had to be pushed around in a wheelchair. Pam carried on looking after her husband and doing everything, not asking for help, doing it all herself.

Her husband became agitated—frustrated at not being able to do things for himself. His moods should have been intolerable, but Pam took it all in her stride. Eventually, it became too much for her. Her husband began to deteriorate and she realised she could not carry on. She decided to find a home for him. He was only in the home for three weeks when he died. She was tearing herself apart with guilt. When Pam admitted this, I relaxed her into a hypnotic state and suggested that she was ready to forgive herself, and to forgive her husband for his bitter attitude to all help she had been trying to give him. Pam's face expressed immense relief.

Pam had four sessions and by the end was a different woman. She now felt she was in control of her life and valued herself in a more positive way. She had learned to let others help her after always being the one to help others (permission was given by the client to report this case history). Pam came to realise during our sessions that no woman is a saint.

Having removed the headache, Pam was convinced that she could be helped. I knew during the conversation we had had that there was a hidden agenda of which Pam was unaware. I challenged her and said:

"You must have hated your husband at the end? He must have been so angry with you, finding himself unable to do the things he had done as a physically fit person. He must have become very frustrated at his situation and may have taken it out on you, and nothing you ever did would have been right?"

Pam denied this at the first session. I continued to work, using a general hypnotic confusion technique within a deeper relaxation, interjecting with metaphor suggestions to help Pam see herself as she wanted to be—free of her anxiety and stress. The suggestions included seeing herself achieving the results she wanted, going outside on her own, being able to go to Bingo and meet people without feeling that the pavement was going to come up and hit her.

On her second session, she came in and sat down and said she had thought about what was said and realised that, yes she had to admit she did begin to hate everything. She resented it so much she could not do anything she wanted to do. It was always for him. That he had died so soon after putting him in a home created enormous guilt.

In helping this client to release her guilt, we used a simplistic technique. We asked her to feel where in the body did the guilt exist? Go into your body and ask permission—will it allow you to receive the healing? She received the answer "Yes". So where do you feel this guilt feeling? She went to straight to the heart area and so we asked her to give a description of what does it look like. Pretend as if like a child. She said, "It is a great black blob." "What texture is it?" She said hard and spiky. Did it have a smell? It smelt of a sewer. Did it have a sound? " A screaming screech", she said. Now she was told:

> "Your body has every resource it needs to heal itself. Just believe. I want you now to ask your body to imagine whatever colour pops into your mind. Let that colour be full of love that will dissolve away this black feeling of guilt."

I watched her, helping her to tune in. After about a minute I asked:

> "Has it changed?" She said,"Yes it is smaller."
> "What does it feel like now?" I asked her.
> "Softer," she said. " It's grey now, not black. The sound is not so high pitched and the texture is softer. The smell is a little sweeter."

I asked her to continue feeling that light and that love flowing all around that part of the body. She continued and after another minute or so she said,

> "It is very small now. It's so small it has no smell, has no touch; it feels more or less airy-fairy."

Then, using hypnotic technique, I said to her,

> "Now make it so small and when I click my fingers it will be gone."

The client moved, the flicker of her eyelids showed it had gone.

She was then asked to allow the colour of love that she had chosen to now spread and fill the void the feeling had left—to feel that colour and love flow right across the whole of her chest, right down through her body and up through her head; to allow the healing process to rejuvenate and regenerate every single cell in her body. This client was in a deep hypnosis state and was allowing her body to enjoy this experience and we asked her to bring it outside herself. Then I brought her back. Her face was glowing, her eyes were shining.

In some cases like this, a client may hallucinate and this particular one saw her husband was there. Pam sensed her husband and asked her husband to forgive her. I then asked her,

> "Can you forgive yourself?"

This was the last healing round. Pam cried with that reaction of joy and relief.

On the third session Pam came again and she said she had been able to go out with her daughter without the pavement coming up to hit her. She had been able to do a lot of things that she had not done before and so we reinforced that she would be able to go out, using her imagination and creating in her mind the places she wanted to go to so that she could create and go in reality. On the fourth session, she said she felt great, explaining what had been happening to her.

She had strong emotions of guilt, did not feel like eating, and felt depressed. Her thoughts went in circles as she blamed herself; she could not think clearly and slept badly. The cycle would continue magnifying the way she felt. She became stressed and worried, and lost weight. Her body was tense and fearful; when out of doors she experienced vertigo. But after this last session, the symptoms disappeared completely.

A stutterer

He was in a very prominent architect, brought up in a wealthy family, given everything he wanted. He had a very strict father and this man found that when he was stressful or met people who reminded him of his father he became anxious and would stutter. He reported that there was an occasion when he was trying to help his dad with DIY and his father shouted:

"Don't do that; can't you do anything properly?"

He found himself stuttering when trying to answer back. From that time on whenever his father or anyone spoke to him in an angry way he stuttered.

After college he joined his father's business. The stuttering was still a problem and it became worse to the point where it became embarrassing. He felt under his father's shadow; he loved his father and never realised why he stuttered. All he wanted was his father's approval. His father was a perfectionist and expected his son to be the same. His father, like any father, was trying to help his son to be better than himself, which is usually what parents hope to do. The belief that he had got to be as good as his father, stopped him from actually achieving his aim.

In therapy he was regressed back to a time as a child, using the Belmont Way. This allowed him to see that little boy, sending love and healing thoughts of forgiveness to the child that he was, and to his father. For the rest of his life he would be able to speak easily and clearly without difficulty.

The therapist suggested that it would help him to breath deeply and slowly, and in hypnosis he was able to relax and speak clearly and easily.

The suggestion to his subconscious mind was that no matter what situation he found himself in, he would be relaxed and completely in control, speaking clearly and easily with no problem at all.

On his second visit the condition had improved tremendously; he was no longer afraid of his father and after two sessions he had stopped stuttering and he felt that he was in control, He was no longer bothered about anyone shouting at him, could speak clearly, easily, and knew that he had the confidence to do what he wanted to do,

Second stutterer

Jeremy did not have a bad stutter; he was slightly dyslexic but whenever he became stressful or upset, he could not stop himself from stuttering, particularly on the telephone or when he had to talk to someone he didn't know. This indicated a problem of his childhood. On an occasion during his first week at school he was asked to stand up and answer questions by the teacher. He felt terrified and could not speak properly. The teacher's attitude made him feel worse and from that time on he was never able to speak in class without stuttering, although he did not stutter at other times. Gradually the situation grew worse and he found himself stuttering whenever he had to talk to someone that he didn't know. Whether or not this situation was responsible for him developing dyslexia is difficult to assess. Using a form of Dave Elman technique, modified to suit a young teenager, he was given direct suggestions that his subconscious mind would change his behaviour in such a way as to ensure that, from this time forward, he would speak easily, calmly and clearly in any situations he encountered. On his second visit, he reported a great improvement not only in his speech, but also in his self-confidence. On the third session, he felt confident that he was in control and didn't need any further treatment.

The neuropeptide system

The sharp edge of neurobiological research is revealing a new understanding of the dichotomy of the mind-body interaction. An integrated communication system between the mind and the endocrine, autonomic and the immune systems is conceived as functioning in the neuropeptide system. In 1985 Doctors Pert, Ruff, Weber and Herkenham, working in the Biochemistry Division of the National Institute of Mental Health, proposed that neuropeptides and their receptors *'function as a previously unrecognised **psychosomatic network**'*. Summarised, this is what they had to say:

> *A major conceptual shift in neuroscience has been wrought by the realization that brain function is modulated by numerous chemicals in addition to classical neurotransmitters. Many of these informational substances are neuropeptides, originally studied in other contexts as hormones, 'gut peptides' or growth factors. Their numbers presently exceed 50 and most, if not all, alter behaviour and mood states, although only endogenous analogs of psychoactive drugs such as morphine, Valium, and phencyclidine have been well appreciated in this context. We now realize that their signal specificy resides in receptors (distinct classes of recognition molecules), rather than the close juxtaposition occurring at classical synapses. Rather, precise brain distribution patterns for many neuropeptides receptors have been determined. A number of brain loci, many within emotion-mediating brain areas, are enriched with many types of neuropeptide receptors, suggesting a convergence of information at these 'nodes'. Additionally, neuropeptide receptors occur on mobile cells of the immune systems; monocytes can chemotax to numerous neuropeptides via processes shown by structure-activity analysis to be mediated by distinct receptors indistinguishable from those found in the brain. Neuropeptides*

and their receptors thus join the brain, glands, and immune system in a network of communication between brain and body, probably representing the biochemical substrate of emotion.

Translated into lay terms, very briefly, this is saying that the mind is able to modify the functioning of the brain in order to bring about physical changes in bodily functions; which is exactly what hypnotherapy is all about—Mind over Matter!

3

What you think is what you are

You are what your subconscious mind thinks that you are, and ever since you were born, your subconscious mind has been constantly modifying its conception of who you are.

Ever since that momentous day when you were forcibly ejected from that dark, warm, cosy environment of the womb, down the birth canal into that cold, bright, noisy world, your subconscious has been building that self-image of the person that you are.

In the beginning all that is in that self-image is the genetic inheritance from both your parents plus, of course, your reaction to the birth experience.

Parental influence

If you are fortunate enough to have well-informed parents who have learnt all they could about the birth experience, then your mother will have practised relaxation and self-hypnosis techniques, which ensure that she has a normal and natural birth with minimum discomfort and as little intervention from the midwifery team as possible. In that case you start life with an enormous advantage over the vast majority of mortals. A traumatic birth experience may leave you psychologically scarred for life. From the moment of your birth and for every moment of your life thereafter, your every experience, or at least, your reaction to every experience, creates changes to that self-image.

Sigmund Freud

In the study of the development of that self-image we are indebted to Sigmund Freud (1858–1939). Before Freud, psychology had concentrated on the study of consciousness. It was Freud who recognised the importance of the subconscious (which he called the unconscious). After gaining his medical degree from the University of Vienna, Freud went on to study with a French psychiatrist, Dr Jean Charcot, who was using hypnosis to treat patients suffering from hysteria.

Subsequently, Freud established a practice as a specialist in nervous disorders and his ideas still form the basis of psychoanalysis. When he established his practice, he was not happy with the conventional methods of the day. He was persuaded by a friend, Dr Josef Breuer, to use hypnosis. Because he found difficulty in inducing hypnosis in all his patients, Freud resorted to encouraging them to talk about their problems. This developed into his technique of 'Free Association of Ideas', which eventually became psychoanalysis. As patients discussed their thoughts and their dreams, they often remembered events of their childhood, which had been repressed by the subconscious. By recalling these experiences, the client was often able to deal with them successfully.

Freud's three-fold structure

Freud believed in a three-fold structure of the personality, the Id, the Ego and the Superego. The Id is the basic drives and instincts with which one is born, and the need to satisfy those needs as quickly and effectively as possible without regard to the effect on others. The Ego, he postulated, is the modifying factor of the Id's desires. It has the job of ensuring that the way in which those desires are satisfied is not detrimental to the personality. The Superego is that aspect of personality which develops as the personality absorbs the standards of behaviour and moral judgements from the parents and its own environment, and eventually develops its own standards of morality and behaviour: its own conscience.

Psychodynamic theories

Personality development is determined by events and conflicts that take place within the mind. Freud believed that the source of all psychosomatic disturbance was in what he called the unconscious; that personality was formed out of the continual struggle between desire to satisfy inborn instincts, such as sex and aggression, while living within an environment that will not tolerate such uninhibited behaviour.

Two colleagues of Freud, Carl Jung and Alfred Adler, held different beliefs from those of Id, Ego, and Superego.

Carl Jung

Carl Jung joined Freud in 1909 and split from him in 1913. He differed from Freud in that he believed that Libido or Psychic Energy was the source of *all* the basic drives, not just the sexual ones and that Libido develops in the ordinary course of the body's metabolism, instead of Freud's megalomaniac Id kept under control by the Ego.

Jung proposed two levels of consciousness: a personal unconscious and a collective unconscious. The personal unconscious contains all the repressed thoughts, memories and experiences of the lifetime from birth onwards and the collective unconscious contains behaviour patterns, instinctive behaviour and race memories handed down through millions of years of evolution.

Alfred Adler

Alfred Adler (1870–1937) left Freud in 1911 to establish his own school. He, like Freud and Jung, believed that unconscious needs and congenital forces condition behaviour, but to Adler they are the social needs, the reactions of a pack instinct. He believed that the driving force is towards Superiority probably engendered by the feelings of Inferiority experienced by every infant during its years of complete dependency on adults for all its needs and which is frequently compounded during childhood, at school, and in the home.

Oral conflicts

Freud studied the human libido in detail and theorised that, in addition to the genital organs, the mouth and the anus could equally be regarded as focus of sexual response. Recognising that emotional problems frequently originate in conflicts in early childhood, Freud suggested that the development of sexuality had passed through three stages of development since birth. Each related to one of these areas. The earliest stage he called the oral stage, the first year, during which sexual response is centred on the mouth. The baby experiences love and comfort during feeding, particularly breast-feeding. Interruption of the feeding or denial of feeding when the infant is hungry can, Freud suggests, cause emotional conflicts which, if not resolved, can predispose the child to a feeling of deprivation, inhibition, or neurotic conditions, aggression and a grasping nature. These he called the oral conflicts. Unresolved oral conflicts, he suggested, cause compulsive behaviour and depressive illness.

Anal conflicts

The second most important stage, according to Freud's theories, is the anal stage, the second and third years. This is the stage during which 'potty training' starts and in which the child may find satisfaction in expelling or retaining faeces; it is often a period of conflict between the mother and the child when he/she would prefer to be cuddled or fed—the child's first encounter with authority. The child begins to learn that reward and punishment are linked to success or failure in controlling bowel functions. Unresolved anal conflicts, he suggests, cause obsessive behaviour, paranoid behaviour and hypochondria and may also result in sado-masochism.

Genital conflicts

Freud's third stage is the genital stage, starting round about third and fourth years of age and continuing until puberty, with a period known as latency—usually after the seventh year and continuing into puberty—when the interest turns to sports, school work, hobbies and forming associations with the peer group and showing lack of interest in sexuality. In the early years of this stage, the child becomes aware of his/her own genital area, plays with and fingers the genitals, and shows interest in the genitals of other children and, in later stages, masturbation. During this stage the child takes a passionate interest in the parent of the opposite sex. Conflicts are created if the parent of the opposite sex rejects the child, and when the child is made to feel guilty about the genital area. According to Freud, unresolved genital conflicts can cause hysteria, anxiety and phobias.

Freud maintains it is during this period that the Oedipus complex in boys and the Electra complex in girls develops, named after the Greek mythology whereby Oedipus killed his father and married his mother. According to Freud, all young boys sexually desire their mother and would like to kill their father out of jealousy, but because they think that their father is aware of this desire, they are afraid of the father. The Electra complex follows more or less the same pattern with girls. These conflicts eventually resolve as the child matures and identifies with the parent of the same sex and enters a latency period when the child bonds more with its own sex, avoiding intimacy with the opposite sex. However, delayed development during the Oedipus and Electra periods may explain some cases of homosexuality.

The physical discomforts relating to or concerned with bodily symptoms accompanying these emotional disturbances are very real. That there are no obvious medical or neurological signs or symptoms does not make the psychosomatic responses any less painful. These problems might almost be said to resemble the reverse side of the 'placebo effect' coin.

On the one hand the mind is creating an illness and on the other it is curing an illness. Whereas we can trace the neural or emotional pathway by which the psychosomatic disturbance has travelled from mind to body, i.e. via the mind modulation of the neuropeptide system, we are still in the dark as to the workings of the 'placebo effect'.

There can be little doubt that what triggers the placebo effect is suggestion. The suggestion need not be vocal, indeed, the most powerful suggestions are frequently completely nonverbal (see *Chapter 1*, p.?). Although the power of suggestion has been known and used for hundreds of years, the concept of the powerful placebo effect was pursued by H K Beecher (*The Powerful Placebo*, 1953). In a careful investigation of 25 studies, he calculated that one third of those being studied improved due to the placebo effect.

A conservative estimate

Many studies claim the placebo effect is much more effective, as much as 60 per cent in some cases, which include cases involving the central nervous system. The placebo effect often proved to be as effective as some recently introduced psychotropic drugs for the treatment of brain disorders and doubts have been raised that some of the new drugs are not as effective as the placebos. Questions have been raised as to whether the results attributed to these new drugs might not also have been due to the placebo effect rather then the psychotropic drugs (Carol Hart, 1999).

However, it is not only in the field of medicinal treatment that the placebo has been proved to be as effective as conventional treatment:

> *'Forty years ago a young Seattle cardiologist named Leonard Cobb conducted a unique trial of a procedure then commonly used for angina, in which doctors made a small incision in the chest and tied knots in two arteries in order to try to increase blood flow to the heart. It was a popular technique—90% of patients reported that it helped—but when Cobb compared it to placebo surgery in which he made the incisions but did not tie off the arteries, the sham operations proved just as successful. The*

procedure, known as internal mammary ligation, was soon abandoned.'

The Placebo Prescription by Margaret Talbot
(*New York Times Magazine*, January, 2000)

Placebo or suggestion

Some psychologists propose that the placebo effect could be due to the very powerful suggestion, accepted by the patient, that the treatment will make them well. The hypnotherapist does not just propose this as a hypothesis, he knows it to be true. In his preliminary chat, every good hypnotherapist will emphasise to the client that the treatment will be effective only if the client genuinely wants it to happen, that all hypnosis is really self-hypnosis and that the client's own subconscious mind is the all-powerful medium which will bring about the changes desired by the client. The question every hypnotherapist must surely ask is, 'What is the difference between the hypnotic suggestion and the placebo, does the hypnotic suggestion trigger the placebo, or are they both the same?'

Placebo or drug

Irving Kirsch, a psychologist at the University of Connecticut, believes that the effectiveness of Prozac® and similar drugs may be attributed almost entirely to the placebo effect. He and Guy Sapirstein analysed nineteen clinical trials of antidepressant drugs and concluded that the *expectation of improvement*, not adjustments in brain chemistry, accounted for 75 per cent of the drugs' effectiveness (Kirsch, 1998). 'The critical factor,' says Kirsch, 'is our beliefs about what is going to happen to us. You don't have to rely on drugs to see profound transformation.' In an earlier study, Sapirstein analysed 39 studies, done between 1974 and 1995, of depressed patients treated with drugs, psychotherapy or a combination of both. He found that 50 per cent of the drug effect was due to the placebo response.

A person's hopes and beliefs about the outcome of a treatment, combined with their own susceptibility to suggestion, may have a significant biochemical effect. Sensory experience and thoughts can affect neurochemistry. The body's neurochemical system affects and is affected by other biochemical systems, including the hormonal and immune systems. Thus, it is consistent with current knowledge that a person's hopeful attitude and beliefs may be very important to their physical well-being and recovery from illness and injury (Pert *et al*, 1985: 820).

Suggestion a killer?

The power of suggestion must not be underestimated, however.

> '*In one of the most reported cases in modern medical literature S Kinkelstein and MG Howard present a case study showing the power of suggestion at work. This involves a controversial substance made from horse's blood, named Krebiozen. A terminally ill patient heard that a new drug was being tested in the hospital where he was lying, not expecting to live. He begged for the new medication and eventually he was given some. Ten days later there was no trace of the tumours, which were as big as oranges that were killing him. He was discharged. Two months later he was back in hospital, his faith shattered by unfavourable press reports of the drug, and his cancer reactivated. A doctor then gave him an injection of pure water, telling him it was a new type of double strength Krebiozen, whereupon the patient recovered even more rapidly than before, and was once again discharged. Two months later he again learned that the American Medical association had declared Krebiozen to be worthless. Within two days of returning to hospital he was dead.*
>
> Finkelstein and Howard(?year?)

Consciousness and the left brain

So what is it that makes hypnotherapy so successful when all else has failed? In hypnotherapy we are taking advantage of the fact that there are differences in the way that the conscious and the subconscious (Freud called it the unconscious) minds function. Like the two hemispheres of the brain, the two aspects of mind have quite different functions. It is these differences which make possible the changes that can be effected in hypnosis,

It is quite impossible to prove without question that such a function as subconscious mind actually does exist. Nevertheless, if we assume for the purpose of achieving our ends, i.e. changing behaviours, that the conscious and the subconscious are separate functions of mind, with different capabilities and different faculties, providing we do our job professionally and proficiently, our clients achieve the outcomes they desire; this assumes that they genuinely do desire such an outcome and there are no secondary inhibitions that might stand in the way of this outcome.

If we accept the finding of many psychological studies—that the conscious mind is the subjective aspect of brain activity responsible for enabling us to cope on a continuing basis with the exigencies of everyday life—perhaps it might be argued that the conscious mind is the subjective function of the brain's left hemisphere, logical, rational and analytical. These are the faculties that enable us to get through each day to the best of our ability. At the end of our day, it is the conscious mind—monitoring our system and recognising a state of relaxation of both body and mind—that switches off most of its functions and, in doing so, permits us to fall asleep. There can be very few who have not experienced a night when the conscious mind has not recognised that 'pre-sleep state' and has not switched off, leaving us to lay awake, our mind remorselessly reiterating the events of the day.

Subconscious and the right brain

The same psychological investigations inform us that the subconscious mind never shuts down. From the time of our birth until the day we die the subconscious mind never sleeps. Even when, to all appearances, we are 'unconscious', perhaps as a result of an accident or under anaesthetic or maybe in a coma, our subconscious mind is still aware. From the day we are born and for every second of our life the subconscious mind records our reactions to all that we experience. It is those reactions which constantly modify the self-image that the subconscious has of the person we are. The person that we are today is the person that our subconscious mind believes that we are. All our behaviours are reflections of that self-image. If we desire to effect changes in those behavioural patterns it is through the subconscious that those changes must be made.

Fact-finding questionnaires submitted by GPs have established without doubt that 80 per cent of the patients visiting their surgeries are suffering from psychosomatic rather than physical problems. Their symptoms are emotional rather than bacterial or viral. Their aches and pains are very real but they are of the mind not the body. Just as we know from psychological and neurological research about the faculties of the left hemisphere of the brain, we also know that the faculties and capabilities of the right brain could be said to be at the opposite end of the spectrum.

Just as the left brain is rational and logical and analytical, the right brain is imaginative, creative, artistic, musical. In other words, whereas the left brain is logical and objective, the right brain is imaginative and subjective. These differences are of prime importance to the hypnotherapist. It is, of course, obvious that even the most right brain person must, in order to function effectively, exercise the left brain faculties. The two hemispheres are connected, just above the place where the spinal column enters the skull, by a huge bundle of nerve fibres called the *Corpus Callosum*. These enable the two hemispheres to work in coordination.

The mysterious subconscious

The history of hypnosis is bedevilled by superstition, witch-craft, sorcery and the fairground sideshows of the nineteenth century. Stories of Mesmer and Rasputin are far better known than the great works of Elliotson, Braid, Esdaile and Coue.

Who has never been 'mesmerised'? Although I, in all ear-nestness and sincerity, tell my clients, 'There is no mystery, sorcery or witchcraft about hypnosis' and say it with a smile so that they know I am joking, I then go on to say, 'We are simply taking advantage of the differences between the way in which the conscious and the subconscious function.'

Nevertheless, I have to admit to myself that I don't really fully understand **how** the subconscious works. We know what it can do and we know how to stimulate it into doing that which we wish it to do. We are rather in the same position as the man of 70 years ago who pressed his brand new electric light switch. I know that if I do the right things it will work but just about how the subconscious works its magic, I have only a glimmer-ing of understanding. I have listened to many who claim to understand fully the workings of the subconscious, but when one analyses what they have said, it all boils down to what that man would have said 70 years ago: 'I know how it works, you press this switch and the light comes on. It's electric.' He might just as well have said 'It's magic'.

It is not many years since Doctors Pert, Ruff, Weber and Herkenham, working at the Biochemistry Division of the National Institute of Mental Health, proposed:

> *'Neuropeptides and their receptors function as a previously unre-cognised psychosomatic network. Neuropeptides and their recep-tors thus join the brain, glands, and immune system in a network of communication between brain and body, probably representing the biochemical substrate of emotion.'*

They have described the circuitry but not how and why it works.

We know why it works but not yet how. We know about the development of the critical faculty in the conscious mind and not in the subconscious. We know this develops at about the age of five or six years. Once that critical faculty develops, we can no longer tell a child any sort of nonsense and have him/her believe it without question: 'A big fat man will come down every chimney in the land and bring presents for every good little boy and girl.'

But the critical faculty develops only in the conscious mind. When direct communication is possible with the subconscious mind, as in hypnosis, then the subconscious will accept suggestions and instructions without question.

The subconscious is immensely powerful. It is capable of initiating change in just about every aspect of a person's behaviour. It has also been shown that, given the correct suggestions in ideal conditions, the subconscious can initiate changes in blood chemistry, blood pressure, and nervous disorders, as well as dealing very successfully with a whole range of psychological problems, such as claustrophobia, anxiety, panic states, depression, lack of confidence and low self-esteem.

What is the issue?

Hypnotherapy works because the technique of hypnotic induction is such that tensions are released and inhibitions are lowered. The relaxation process itself is sufficient to achieve this in many cases even without inducing hypnosis. However, it very often proves to be the case that the client does not know what the problem really is. The presenting of a case of low self-esteem is frequently just the outward presentation of a very deep issue originating in early childhood, or possibly the first cause was a teenage sexual assault or even nothing worse than the deep embarrassment of a young child being chastised in front of the class for wetting her knickers. It may take a couple of sessions of regression to childhood to enable the client to become capable of revealing these traumas. Hypnotherapy techniques enable the practitioner to identify the prime cause quickly and painlessly (using disassociation techniques). Very often the issue which the client thinks was the prime cause was not the case. Accurate diagnosis is probably the most powerful tool in hypnotherapy's toolbox. Once the source of the original trauma is established, direct or indirect suggestion under hypnosis will, in most cases, achieve the desired outcome.

What happens next?

Achieving a successful outcome of the client's problem or problems depends almost entirely on overcoming his/her anxiety about hypnosis and establishing a belief in the hypnotherapist's ability to help. In the client's mind are the questions 'What is he/she going to do?' 'What's it like?'

Giving the client a full explanation of the way hypnotherapy works in simple words and explaining in detail the technique one is about to employ will reduce or completely remove the anxiety and, by doing this with empathy and understanding, the success of the session is almost certainly guaranteed. If the client is convinced in this preliminary chat that the hypnotherapy will be successful, then it almost certainly will be. The first few minutes are the most critical; they herald success or failure.

Right or left brain?

There are many factors involved in a successful hypnotherapy outcome and one is whether the client is right brain dominant or left brain dominant. We know the faculties of the two hemispheres and we know that a left brain dominant person will react quite differently to every situation from a right brain dominant person. Whereas a left brain person will approach a decision-making situation by carefully weighing the pros and cons before taking the next rational and logical step, the right brain person is very likely to assess the situation from an emotional viewpoint and make the decision intuitively. Of the two types, the left brain person will be the more difficult to deal with. The left brain person tends to lack imagination and has problems with visualisation; both of these faculties are of great value in the hypnotherapy process.

If, in the preliminary chat, the hypnotherapist has convinced the right brain dominant client that hypnotherapy will
work for him/her, and that the hypnotherapist has the skill
and experience to make it work, the client will relax and 'go
with it'. The outcome will invariably be successful. However,
the left brain dominant person, while accepting all that the
hypnotherapist is saying, will, during the induction, be criti-
cally analysing what is being said and how it is being said, what
is happening and what is going to happen, and whether it is
working or not working, instead of just relaxing and 'going
with the flow'.

The problem presented by the dichotomy of the brain can
most easily be resolved by using suitable inductions in either
case. In the first instance, it is necessary to know with which
type of brain we are dealing. This can be assessed by using an
appropriate suggestibility test. The 'lemon test' (see p.65) is
one such test. It is preferred because it tests the imagination
and the ability to visualise through all five senses, and is an
excellent indicator of the strength of the brain's right or left
bias.

Experience suggests that a left brain type will respond
better to a long slow physical relaxation type of induction,
probably with low, soft music in the background, whereas the
right brain type will respond well to an Elman induction which
demands a good imagination and visualisation.

The hypnotherapist's responsibility

There is probably no more succinct way of expressing the therapist's philosophy than with the words, 'Do as you would be
done by'. The therapist, particularly the hypnotherapist, is in a
position of heavy responsibility when he/she accepts the commitment to enabling clients resolve issues that are presented.
While it is never possible to guarantee 100 per cent success,
nevertheless, the hypnotherapist will expect him or herself to
deliver just that and will be disappointed if this outcome is not
realised. No matter how simple or complex the issue may be, it
makes no difference to the hypnotherapist's approach or to
the total focus of his/her attention. Whether it is a simple case

of stopping smoking or nail biting, or a complex case of lack of confidence, anxiety, depression, panic states, agoraphobia or stress, to the client it is a matter of supreme importance.

The last resort

In nearly every instance, it is a question of 'the last resort'. That smoker may be a sufferer from emphysema. Stopping smoking will extend his life expectancy and such is the benefit to the client. The benefit to the hypnotherapist is beyond price. There is no feeling of satisfaction greater than the happy smile and the heart-felt 'Thank you for your help' as the client leaves for the last time.

The hypnotherapist never stops learning. Every client teaches us something. No two clients react in exactly the same way to the same induction. It is impossible not to be fascinated by the study of the human mind and the countless variables in emotional responses. The hypnotherapist is like a detective—constantly searching for clues behind the words, reactions and body language. Signs and symptoms can frequently tell a very different story from that presented by the client. The middle aged man with low self-esteem might well be suffering from the effects of an acute embarrassment, experienced as a result of a wet bed at boarding school. The well-qualified hypnotherapist with a sincere desire to help can do more than most to make a change.

Responsibility

Not only must the qualified hypnotherapist do all in his/her power to help the client to the best of his/her ability, there is an additional responsibility to conduct one's self in a manner both ethical and professional in order to protect the reputation of the profession as a whole. All professional teaching establishments have a duty to maintain adequate Codes of Practice and Ethical Standards. While standards of behaviour, care and treatment in many caring professions appear to be below what the public is entitled to expect, hypnotherapy has a much better record in this respect than any other. It is incumbent upon all practitioners to ensure that this high standard is maintained.

Deceptive symptoms

Physical symptoms often mask a serious case of chronic stress which, if allowed to continue, could lead to hypertension (high blood pressure), strokes, heart disease or, many doctors believe, cancer.

Reggie, a rather short man, middle-aged, anxious looking, complained of painful joints and constant stomach pains. He was slightly bent, typical of long-standing stomach pain. In addition to the joint pains, he frequently suffered severe headaches. His symptoms were seriously affecting his ability to do his job. His doctor had been unable to find any physical cause for his ailments and had referred him to a specialist, but the specialist could find no organic disorder to explain the symptoms. The problem had been getting worse over the past two years. A family friend had suggested hypnotherapy.

Asked about his job, he explained that he worked for a finance company and was employed to visit people who were in default with their hire purchase payments on their cars. His job was to get payment or take possession of the car keys and drive the car away. An extremely stressful job. He had to take a lot of verbal abuse and frequently threats of physical abuse. He admitted that every house call was a cause for anxiety. Every day he anticipated that this might be the day when he would meet a drug addict on a bad trip.

In view of his state of anxiety and the fact that he had had some difficulty with the 'lemon test', a physical relaxation induction was preferred. Reggie responded well and went into deep trance without difficulty. Reggie had three sessions. Suggestions of ego boosting, confidence and relaxation, including 'As you approach every house door you feel confident, relaxed and completely at ease, feeling confident that you can deal with every situation that occurs', were reiterated at each session. By the third session he was completely free of the symptoms and ready to resume work. A follow-up three months later found him doing his job without problems and very happy with the outcome. His physical symptoms had completely disappeared.

June's colostomy

June had to have an operation for a colostomy. She was a very nervous woman, extremely anxious to please everyone. She was very thin and also fussy about what she ate. On discussing how we could help her, June revealed a belief she had that she could not eat cheese or bananas. She was not eating properly at all and omitting quite a few foods necessary to sustain a healthy body. At first she thought she might be anorexic but was not.

Her fear began when she had trouble with her bowels. She was not having a proper bowel movement, due to not eating the correct foods to help alleviate this problem. She was a hard worker and a perfectionist. When she did eat foods that she thought were not good for her, she would get upset. She was highly stressed when she reached the decision to see a hypnotherapist.

The technique suggested for June was to first explain what hypnosis is and what it is not, gaining a rapport, and answering any questions about the technique or concerns she may have about her health. She was taught to relax, with suggestions that she would be able to instruct her subconscious mind to allow her to use the bathroom at appropriate times, with no side effects or ill effects. On the first session she was able to close her eyes and ask her body for permission to eat the foods that she thought she could not eat. On asking her body permission, she was then asked to visualise the belief that she could eat cheese; she visualised asking herself to eat cheese and the answer she got was that she could do so.

She asked her body what kind of cheese could she eat that would be healthy for her and got the reply 'goat's cheese and cottage cheese'. When she opened her eyes, she looked surprised. She then asked her body if she could eat fruit. This process went on, in the same way, asking 'can I eat X or Y?', and if the answer was yes, what kind of fruit. A banana came to mind. She had believed she could not eat bananas: this process continued. The suggestion was made that she asked her body before she prepared any food if what she was planning to eat would be all right for that meal. This exercise was given to her to go home and practise, and eat what her body said she could eat.

At the second session, she was very excited and said she found the exercise very useful; she had felt calmer and more in control of herself and her bowels, and had suffered no discomfort during the week. The effect of these three sessions was that she felt so well, she never had a colostomy and the bowel was working in such a way that she felt herself in control. She felt much calmer and more relaxed generally, and the relaxation during the sessions had helped her to be less stressed in situations that, in the past, would have made her very anxious. The key to her success was that she now felt in control.

Under certain circumstances, this technique could work not only with food problems, but also with other issues that are emotionally linked, for example taking tablets, medicine, drinking liquids, encouraging patients to believe that they do have control of their bodies. In some circumstances teaching patients to relax will help change their beliefs about themselves. Understanding the personalities and the type of person one is dealing with helps to suggest which technique will be best for the client/patient; most nurse carers are taught to empathise and understand the patients through their own training.

Using hypnosis, a simple technique for helping a client to stop them panicking is to teach them to breathe—a useful technique which is easy to teach.

Breathing exercise one

First tell the person to take a deep breath for a count of three, hold the breath to a count three, let the breath out to a count of three, and then hold for a count of three. Repeat this two or three times, or even more, until the person is calm. This stimulates and fills the brain with oxygen; lack of oxygen creates the panic feelings.

Breathing exercise two

Place your hands on your lap palms down, close your eyes, and imagine that you are breathing in through your hands: as you breathe in, through your hands, up through your arms, right up to your head; as you breathe out, back down the back of your back, right the way down to your feet, breathing up round again, back up to your hands. Repeat this as many times as you feel comfortable. As you breathe feel yourself letting go, breathing out all your tensions.

Introduced by Robin Hook

Practising this exercise will help the client or patient to relax quite easily.

Using a direct command example

> If someone is in pain, or has just had an accident, by saying to him or her in a confident manner:
>
> *'The pain will stop hurting in one minute.'*

The words used can be beneficial in reassuring a person on a subconscious level and to be aware of the language used in front of a person in pain can help alleviate some of the discomfort. When training a therapist to learn to listen, especially in hypnotherapy, it is the language used that encourages the client to gain the results they are seeking. Learn how to listen to the words people say and how to respond in a way that lets them know you have heard.

4

Treatment of medical disorders

Hypnotherapy has been proved to be of benefit for many conditions including gastrointestinal problems, such as irritable bowel syndrome and Crohn's disease; stomach ulcers and ulcerative colitis have all responded to treatment under hypnosis (Klien and Spiegel, 1989). It was demonstrated in controlled conditions that, compared with patients who had received no hypnotherapy, there was a 39 per cent reduction in basal acid output in those cases where hypnotherapy was given.

Incidence of relapse

When studying the incidence of relapse in duodenal ulcer patients in a one-year controlled follow-up, it was found that 100 per cent of those who received medication until the condition cleared up had suffered relapse whereas, in exactly the same conditions, of those who had received hypnotherapy only 53 per cent relapsed (Colgan *et al*, 1988).

There have been many investigations into the efficacy of hypnotherapy in the treatment of irritable bowel syndrome. Probably the most prolific worker in this field is Dr Peter Whorwell of Manchester who has published papers on the subject since 1997. He insists that targeting suggestions on gut activity is a far superior technique than the use of general suggestions of relaxation alone. With twenty years experience in the practice of hypnotherapy I found this to be the case in almost every type of treatment. The finer the focus of attention, for example in cases such as smoking, drinking, weight loss and phobias, suggestions implanted into the subconscious mind are more effective.

In book after book, hypnotists have quoted cases of successful treatment of 'untreatable' conditions. When asked to comment on these cases the most frequent response from the British Medical Association was 'spontaneous regression' or 'inaccurate diagnosis'. In other words, 'It wasn't cured because it didn't exist in the first case' or 'It would have got better anyway, without being treated.'

The unbalanced mind

Strangely, everybody, from the specialist consultant down to the man in the street, easily accepts that the mind is able to create or acerbate disease—'Oh yes, he's a nervous type you know. When he gets a bit of stress his eczema/asthma/psoriasis/ulcer, plays up'—but they find it difficult to accept that what the mind can damage it can also restore. Every doctor, every psychologist and most well-read lay people are aware of such problems as hysterical paralysis, hysterical blindness and hysterical dumbness or deafness. In many cases, the medical profession has no answers for these people. The vast majority can be successfully treated by hypnosis. All these conditions are aberrations of the mind. All that is required is the correct suggestion implanted into the subconscious mind and the condition is cured. Only in hypnosis is it possible to access the subconscious. This, of course, is an over-simplification, but nevertheless is quite true. Conditions must be conducive, the hypnotherapist must be skilful, and the patient must be co-operative.

A question of confidence

The patient must believe that the therapist can do what he says he can do. That belief must be solid before hypnosis induction is even considered. The initial preliminary casual chat is absolutely critical. From the moment of the first telephone inquiry to the time when the treatment is successfully concluded that preliminary chat is the most vital part of the whole process. During that time, without even mentioning the patient's condition, the treatment proposed, the anticipated outcome, or the hypnotherapist's experience, the patient must become totally convinced of the therapist's ability to produce the desired outcome. And that conviction must come without one word of persuasion from the therapist.

With few exceptions, every patient visiting a hypnotist for the first time suffers anxiety on many accounts. Hypnosis is a journey into the unknown. Every other avenue has been explored, but none has proved of benefit. Can this mysterious hypnosis thing really work? What's going to happen? Can he take over my mind? Will he make me say things I don't want to say? What if I can't be hypnotised, where do I go from here?

Absence of doubt = success

There must not be the slightest doubt in the hypnotist's mind that he/she can enable the desired outcome. Even the tiniest shadow of doubt will be instantly conveyed to the patient, i.e. the tone of voice on the telephone, the manner of greeting as they meet, the demeanour of the hypnotherapist as the initial formalities (name, address, phone number etc.) are completed. The patient's sensitivity, heightened by anxiety, is registering every nuance of the hypnotherapist's behaviour. The slightest anomaly can in a moment destroy the patient's already shaky confidence. Success or failure is so finely balanced. In that fraction of a second the success of the session is threatened.

Suggestion is incredibly powerful. If all goes well and everything meets the patient's concept of what to expect and his/her impression of the therapist is favourable, then suggestion will be accepted and the success of the session is almost guaranteed (see Chapter 1, the civil servant).

Suggestion plus imagination

If the most powerful weapon in our armoury is suggestion, then the next must be imagination—the patient's imagination. Without imagination we have little chance of success.

Once the initial 'casual' chat is over, the most important thing the therapist needs to know is the strength of the patient's imagination. A simple suggestibility test will establish this without difficulty. An excellent example of a very effective suggestibility test which can tell us far more than even the most perceptive patient is likely to recognise is the 'lemon test'.

The patient is seated in a comfortable chair, feet flat on the floor. Hands on the lap, seated well back in the chair, eyes closed.

'Imagine yourself in a room in our own home. It doesn't matter which room.

Look around the room, remind yourself what it looks like.

Now go into the kitchen. Look around the kitchen, remind yourself what the kitchen looks like.

Now stand in front of the work surface and on a suitable chopping board see a lemon and a sharp knife.

Look closely at the lemon. See the pores in the peel of the lemon.

Holding the lemon firmly in one hand, take the knife in the other hand and slice the lemon in half.

Look, now, at the cut surface of the lemon. See the juice on the cut surface.

The hand that is holding the lemon now lifts it to your mouth.

You lick the cut surface of the lemon.

Now put the lemon back down on the chopping board, and open your eyes.

If the patient has successfully completed the whole of this test without difficulty then you have tested all aspects of his/her capability of visualisation. You have tested the ability to see, to touch, to feel, to smell and to taste. You have identified a very right brain person and one who will, all other things being favourable, respond very well to suggestion under hypnosis.

The above technique is not infallible. No technique can be called infallible when one is dealing with the human mind.

The mind is so infinite in its variety, it would be impossible to unequivocally state that anything is infallible

A man came to see me because he wanted to overcome a very heavy smoking habit. He reported that he generally smoked 40 cigarettes a day but often far exceeded this when under pressure at work. He was a professional engineer with very heavy responsibilities for public safety on the very large projects of which he was in charge. He was experiencing breathing difficulties and his doctor diagnosed emphysema and insisted that he stop smoking.

I took him through the lemon test and he had difficulty with some aspects of the test and I decided that he could well be a left brain type and might not respond very well to the Elman technique which would have been the technique of choice if I had found him to be 'right brain'. I decided to use a slow physical relaxation induction with music playing very quietly in the background. I use this method because it does not, to any great extent, demand the use of visualisation.

He relaxed well and went into hypnosis without any problem. In view of the type of mind I was dealing with I deepened him several times and then gave the instructions to his subconscious mind to make the changes in his behaviour that would ensure that he was a non-smoker from the moment I told him to wake up again. I always give two sessions for smoking. When he came for his second session he had not smoked and had felt no need, nor any desire for cigarettes. I normally use the same induction for both sessions but on this occasion I decided to vary my usual procedure. As an experiment I used the Elman technique, which I never use on left brain types. He relaxed easily and went into a deep state very quickly. When I brought him out of hypnosis he said that he felt as though he had been even deeper than first session. You never can tell!

A blueprint of your life

A question that frequently occupies a patient's mind when they are told that the subconscious mind will effect the changes required of it is, 'What makes us so sure that the subconscious can, or will, make those changes possible?'

This is a question that must be answered even when it has not been asked. Patients frequently have questions in their minds that they, for one reason or another, do not ask. It is the therapist's job to anticipate these questions. By doing so we further bolster their confidence in the hypnotherapist's ability to resolve their problems.

The genetic inheritance

So, what is the answer. From the time we are born our subconscious mind has a 'self-image' of the person we are. When we are born there is only our genetic inheritance in that self-image but whatever we experience, or rather, the way we react to those experiences, from that time on, constantly modifies our self image. We are the person we are today because of what the subconscious mind believes we are. If we wish to make changes in the way we behave, consciously or unconsciously, voluntarily or involuntarily, those changes must be made through the subconscious mind. The subconscious is all-powerful in effecting behavioural change through mind modulation of the neuropeptide system. In this context, behaviour refers to physical as well as emotional responses to environmental influences.

The critical faculty

But this does not explain why one person's subconscious should accept instructions and/or suggestions from another person without question. The reason for this is due to another difference between conscious and subconscious. As every parent will know, up to the age of about five years, or perhaps even earlier, one can tell a child any sort of nonsense and they will believe it without question: 'A big fat man will come down our chimney with a sack on his back and leave your Christmas presents at the foot of your bed and he will do that for every little boy and girl in the world on Christmas Eve.'

But there comes a time when instead of believing everything they are told without question, they begin to question everything. This is because the child is developing a 'critical faculty'. This critical faculty develops only in the conscious mind, never in the subconscious. Thus, if we speak directly to the subconscious instead of going through our conscious mind, the subconscious has no option but to accept what it is told. When the client is in hypnosis we speak directly to the subconscious.

A suitably edited and abbreviated version of the above will serve to answer that question. Of course, in normal everyday living everything we experience we experience in a state of full consciousness. The conscious mind is able to exercise its critical faculty and decide whether a thing is good or bad and whether we like it or not, and whether we believe it or not, before that thing is passed to the subconscious for permanent storage.

Not what it seems

It is not uncommon for the symptoms described by the patient to be a camouflage for a deep-seated issue which has been suppressed for many years. Marie was a lady in her mid-40s, still very good looking with a youthful figure. She complained of lack of confidence and low self-esteem. She had difficulty dealing with people in a one-to-one situation and she wanted to stop biting her nails. She owned a café in the High Street. Her husband had his own building business. There were no children. Both businesses were prosperous. No money worries. But she was a deeply unhappy lady. During a lengthy discussion of her difficulties, it was evident that there was something relating to the marriage that she was not saying. Suggestions were given that at the next session she would achieve deeper levels of relaxation.

Celibate

At the second session she was able to talk about her marriage, but with difficulty. She loved her husband, had married for the first time at 40 and found herself to be frigid. At the first sexual approach from her new husband she froze. It is hard to imagine the strain that couple endured, but they had stayed together. The marriage had never been consummated. Her husband had been very understanding but insistent that she should seek help.

Using the Elman eye closure (Elman, 19??) I took her into light trance and told her that her subconscious mind would know what had been the cause of the frigidity and she would now go back into her childhood to whatever it was that had caused the problem. She went back to age eleven years. The story was very disjointed. She was very emotional and abreacted several times. For brevity and clarity this is the story as it happened.

Her mother had a job in a factory some miles from her home. The firm provided transport—a van fitted with seats. Several women living in the same council estate worked for the same firm and the van went from door to door collecting the women and taking them to work. The same thing worked in reverse at home time. The little girl often went along for the ride on the morning run; the driver would take her back home in time for school. The women rode in the back of the van but the child rode in the cab with the driver. One day as she was playing in the road after school she saw the van. The driver stopped and asked her if she would like a ride as he was going to pick up the women from the factory. En route to the factory he stopped, took the child into the back of the van and raped her. He threatened her with all sorts of terrible things if she ever told anybody. Although she was very distressed and there was blood on her clothing, her mother ignored the whole thing. She must have known what had happened but she took no action. She knew that the driver was a drinking pal of the boss. The child was too frightened to speak. Now, in her 40s, was the first time she had told a soul. All her life she had felt that everybody who looked at her knew. She felt despoiled, guilty, ashamed and unworthy.

Without deepening the trance state, she was told that her subconscious mind would now remove all those negative thoughts and that those feelings of guilt and shame were things of the past, that she wouldn't even think of them ever again. From the time she was told to wake up again she would feel good about herself. She was strong and confident in all those situations that had been difficult for her in the past. Those situations would not ever bother her again. She was happy and relaxed and that feeling would stay with her, day by day getting better and better. Her relationship with her husband would improve day by day and within seven days time she would enjoy a full sexual relationship with her husband.

On her next visit, a week later, in her own words she reported 'When I left last week I felt fantastic. I just couldn't stop smiling. It's been brilliant in the café I felt so good with people. No problem.'

She hesitated, blushing.

'John and I are really man and wife at last. Thank you for giving us back our marriage.'

The jealous wife

Probably the most destructive emotion in any relationship is jealousy. Daphne was in her late 40s. She gave permission for her name to be used. She loved her husband dearly and he returned her love, but her jealousy was destroying their marriage. Theirs was one of many similar stories. There was the six foot, fifteen stone building worker, who was so jealous that when he thought a man, who was sitting several tables away in a café, was looking at his wife, he went across and assaulted him, overturning the table and picking up a heavy chair to use as a weapon. Fortunately he was restrained before he could do more harm. And there was the man who was having an affair with his friend's wife. They were in her bedroom when he became suspicious that she was sleeping with her own husband. Knowing that the husband kept a shotgun in the wardrobe, he took it and fired both barrels at his lover. The result was a very large hole in the headboard and a very frightened wife. The story she told her husband to explain the disappearance of the headboard was weird.

Destructive jealousy

There was no physical violence in Daphne's story. Verbal assaults were, however, not uncommon. Both Daphne and her loving husband were desperately unhappy about Daphne's problem but Daphne could not help herself. She loved her husband and knew that he loved her. The situation was affecting her health and that of her husband. Her jealousy was so extreme that if they were watching television and a pretty woman was shown on the screen she would accuse her husband of lusting after the woman and she would switch off the set. They very seldom watched television. Also, they very seldom went out. What made things even worse was that they owned a hotel in a holiday resort, so they were together all day every day. Her husband never mixed with the guests.

In view of Daphne's distress a slow relaxation induction seemed more appropriate, deepened several times to a deep trance. She was reassured that her husband loved her, that no other woman was any threat to her, no matter where they went; even if pretty women were present she would feel totally secure in his love for her. She had no cause to feel jealousy at any time. A few weeks after her third session she wrote: 'I wanted to tell you of my feelings, after only three sessions I have had with you. After five years of constant fear and the pain of intense jealousy, I had forgotten how to laugh and enjoy life. I was so desperate when I came to see you. From my first session I have been feeling so unbelievably different. I can hardly believe it possible.'

Unfortunately, all those years of 'fear and pain' exacted their toll. Three years later Daphne developed cancer and six months later she died. Investigations have shown that a significant number of cancer sufferers have experienced chronic stress within a two- to three-year period of the cancer developing. Daphne's husband affirmed that those last three years were the happiest of their lives.

Childhood trauma

A high percentage of phobias, obsessions, anxiety states, depression, compulsions and other psychosomatic conditions are the direct result of unresolved childhood traumas. The adult who has a fear of lifts and other enclosed spaces, including aeroplanes, has often been confined in a dark space as a child, or perhaps simply crying for help in the middle of the night when waking from a bad dream, but not being heard by the parents. Or, the worst scenario, being locked in an under the stairs cupboard as punishment for being naughty.

The lost child

A child out shopping with parents in a busy store, perhaps on holiday on the beach, or in a busy fairground, wanders away from the parents in a moment when the attention of the parents is distracted. Suddenly the child looks around and realises that those trousered legs are not Daddy's legs and that skirt is not Mummy's skirt. Instant panic. Even though it may be only a few minutes before child and parents are re-united, the damage is done. The seeds of agoraphobia are sown. In years to come that child may be incapable of leaving its own front door.

Siblings at risk

Judith was a tall and slim twenty 21-year-old attractive young woman. Dark blonde with very long hair, oval features with a wide forehead, she could have been more than just attractive except for her complexion, which was pale and rather greasy with lots of tiny red spots on her forehead. She complained of lack of confidence and a constant feeling of anxiety, and difficulty in dealing with people and busy places.

Judith came as a result of a recommendation from a friend who had similar problems and came for help some two or three years previously. She was obviously very stressed and nervous, sitting on the edge of the seat, leaning forward, hands clasped between her knees.

In the course of 'history taking' it transpired that her mother was 'a bit of an anxious sort of person' but father was 'a strong character and very calm type'. Her relationship with both parents was 'OK'. Questioned about the onset of her problems, she couldn't remember when it all started. Asked to think of a time when they didn't exist, she suggested it could have been about the age of nine but she could not think of anything that happened at about that time which might have been significant. After a lengthy chat about schooldays and her relationship with school friends during which she relaxed considerably, she mentioned having had eating disorders, always feeling fat, not being able to eat in front of others.

There was, I was sure, an issue which she was not yet ready to talk about. In view of her level of anxiety I decide to use a slow physical relaxation followed by a visualisation induction. She responded well to suggestions of calm, confidence and self-esteem.

Deeper waters

At the second session, four days later, she reported having felt much better, but still felt panic when approaching the pub that she regularly visited with her friends. She explained that she always had a couple of glasses of wine before going out with friends in the evening because it was the only way she could feel comfortable but when her friends decided to go to another pub, which was larger and noisier than the small quiet pub that they usually used, she felt such panic that she had run out in tears. She always felt that people were looking at her and thinking that she was so fat. On one occasion when she was out with friends she was wearing a skirt, something she very seldom did; the skirt was not particularly short, just above the knees, but one of her friends shouted 'Oh Judith, we can all see your cellulite.' She was so upset, she ran away home and cried until three o'clock in the morning.

There was obviously some deep-seated issue which she was guarding because it was too painful to recall. I asked her what was her very earliest childhood memory. She went very pale. Sitting on the edge of the seat once again, hands between her knees, clasped tight, head bowed, shaking from side to side. 'No, I can't tell you. No, I can't.' We sat in silence for several minutes before I tried to coax her to speak. At last she appeared to be trying to speak but it seemed that she just could not bring the words out. It took several minutes of stuttering and stammering. Starting and then stopping, eventually she managed to tell me. They had been playing hide and seek. She was about three years old, her brother was three years older. They hid in a space behind the big settee and the wall. She found it impossible to actually say the words but what she was indicating was that he molested her sexually, stripping her naked. This was the first of a sequence of such attacks. At the age of five they were both in her bedroom playing a board game when he did it again. Her mother came into the room and found them both naked. There was a big row and he promised not to do it again.

On another occasion they were in the back seat of the car. It was a long journey, her mother had covered them with a duvet so they could sleep. She was nine. Her brother made her masturbate him under the cover of the duvet. She insisted that she always tried to resist him but he was a strong boy and she didn't want to get him into trouble, although she knew it was wrong and it made her feel very bad.

When she was fifteen, he came into her room and tried to have full sex but she fought him off and she thinks she must have cried out, because her mother burst into the room and caught him. Her father heard the row and came into the room. What went on between the boy and his father she never knew but he was made to apologise to Judith and promise that it would never happen again. That was the last time he tried anything.

Judith was very upset after talking about these experiences but she said she felt a great relief—it was the first time she had told anyone.

She started talking once again about feeling fat but this was a strange form of the problem. She not only felt that she was fat (she wasn't), she felt as though the fat was outside her body. It was as though there was a sort of cobweb of fat all over her body. It was so bad that she sometimes took a pair of scissors and tried to cut the fat from her skin but when she accidentally cut the skin it hurt so she stopped. But then when it felt bad again she would again try and cut it off.

By the time that we had discussed these issues, she was obviously feeling much more at ease and I decided to use a modified Elman technique. She responded very well and achieved a very deep trance. I suggested that her subconscious mind would erase the effects of her childhood experiences and enable her to make a fresh start, free from the problems that had been caused by those experiences. On her third session she was on top of the world. She had been to a restaurant and enjoyed a meal and had visited a strange pub on both occasions without having a glass of wine beforehand and with no problem on either occasion. She had two further sessions just to ensure that the changes were stable. There is no greater reward than the look on the client's face as they take your hand and say, 'Thank you for your help'.

Low spirits can depress

There is often some confusion about the condition described as depression. To most people depression means that a person is feeling in low spirits because things are not going well for them. This condition rarely lasts very long and is effectively cured as soon as things improve. Sometimes, however, the symptoms develop without any apparent cause and can progress to the state when the sufferers require medical help; these are often referred to as being clinically depressed. Around 2 per cent of the population are in this category each year and recent research suggests that women are particularly vulnerable between the ages of twenty to 45 years, especially post natal and in bereavement. Extreme states of depression can descend into neurosis and are frequently accompanied by

Free Floating Anxiety. Depression and anxiety neurosis is by far the most common form of neurosis. Recurrent severe depression can develop into psychosis.

A dangerous confusion

'Never judge a book by its cover.' We all know what we mean by this and by 'The proof of the pudding is in the eating'. Both of these old sayings had great significance where George (not his real name) was concerned. A tall, well-built, pleasant looking man, with dark hair, pale complexion and blue eyes. He was diagnosed as clinically depressed and was initially prescribed Lithium, 75mg twice daily. This was said to have subsequently been changed to 400mg Prothiaden twice daily during the past year. This seems an unbelievably high dosage and is probably wrong. (??I have checked the BNF and he could have been prescribed 400mg of Lithium and 75mg of Prothiaden??vmm)

The week before coming for hypnotherapy, he had been ejected from the family home, which was owned by his wife, after months of violent behaviour. He returned the next day and entered the house and set fire to it. The firefighters found a large kitchen knife hidden behind a chest of drawers in the bedroom.

During a course of twelve sessions (very unusual but this was an unusual case), physical relaxation was followed by deepening via a flight of marble steps into a large garden. This deepening suited George. As he walked slowly down the steps and the long garden path towards a shady lake, on which he could see a pair of swans followed by half a dozen cygnets gliding across the water, he relaxed very well.

Regression to childhood revealed a history of depression from an early age. George had been in a state of depression for as long as he could remember. His mother was a depressive, and his father was one of those men who felt incapable of demonstrating affection.

George felt that his mother didn't want him and his father didn't like him. He made no friends at school. Unhappy at home, he remembers frequent tantrums with his mother. He had several periods in hospital, one of six months—pneumonia, bronchitis, fever and constant coughing. Probably all due to a weak immune system caused by long-term depression.

George had some very unpleasant dreams, not repetitive but of a similar nature. Typically, he was in a large boat with lots of people all dressed in brown. The deck of the boat was covered with shellfish that crunched horribly under his feet. As they broke they gave off a horrible smell which made him feel nauseous—obviously a metaphor for the way he felt about his life. Each session started with a long period of relaxation during which nothing was said but occasional suggestions of 'Deeper, now, so happy now' were made, accompanied by a finger snap. This was followed by suggestions of increased self-confidence and greater self-esteem. After four weeks of very gradual improvement, he reported, 'Not too bad this week, only one bad day'.

After week six, he had an appointment with his psychiatrist (who had agreed to the treatment). The psychiatrist reduced his medication from 400mg to 50mg. By session nine, George assessed himself on a scale of one to ten as 8/10. On reviewing the treatment, it was concluded that the prolonged relaxation was probably the most effective and beneficial aspect of the therapy.

Unhappy families

Such are the advances in medicine, surgery and pharmaceutics that, if we are taken ill these days, we have high expectations of a full recovery after treatment from, or through, our doctor. There are, however, some sufferers for whom medical science does not yet have answers. Their problems are just as serious, if not more serious, than the average, run-of-the-mill health issues that account for the majority of visits to GPs' surgeries. They affect the health and well-being of whole families. They are the addicts. The most common addiction, apart from smoking, is alcohol with gambling a close second and hard drugs not far behind. But there are many people who are

addicted to less dangerous substances that can be just as difficult to control. Chocolate, coffee, and sugar are the common-
est examples. Medical science has nothing to offer these
people; hypnotherapy can put them in control.

A military man

Stan (an ex-sergeant major in the army) had been, in his own
words, 'An alcoholic for a number of years'. He was accompanied by his wife, who reported that she had to search the house
every day to find the bottles of gin or vodka that she knew
would be hidden somewhere but she seldom succeeded in
finding them all. Stan had been to AA but that had not helped.
He had also tried a revulsion treatment. That didn't work
either. She loved her husband and he loved her but the marriage was falling apart. As is so often the case, hypnotherapy
was a last resort. It was agreed that Stan would always have his
wife with him when he attended for therapy—it is never wise to
accept what an alcoholic says about his drinking! Stan had
three sessions. He stopped drinking after the first session. In a
letter three years later he wrote, 'I have not drunk a drop for
over three years. It's good to be happy and a family man
again.'

A disastrous outcome

Not all endings are happy ones. Paul was a drug addict and an
alcoholic. He had been in hospital several times due to injuries
received during drunken escapades. He had on one occasion
jumped off a cliff because he thought he could fly. He had a
big scar in the shape of a cross on his chest. It was self-inflicted.
His family were in despair. When sober he was distraught with
guilt.

Paul started therapy on the understanding that at no time
would he have therapy unless he was sober and 'clean' (i.e. not
on drugs). He had four sessions, each time being taken very
deep, using eye closure, the lift (see p.90) and steps into the
garden. Addicts often prove to be very good subjects. Paul was
one of those—he was a somnambulist. In each session he was

told 'You are a non-drinker and a non-user for the rest of your life and you feel proud of yourself.'

After the fourth session he had been sober and 'clean' for three weeks. He felt confident that he was in control. Two or three weeks later he got a job as gardener/handyman at a local convent. He was so proud and happy, it was the first job he had ever had. His family held a party to celebrate. Some weeks after he started, the man in charge of the maintenance staff left and was replaced by an ex-army colonel. A couple of months after the colonel took over Paul hurt his back while wheeling a too heavy wheelbarrow (his back had been weak ever since his fall from the cliff). When Paul had been off work for a couple of weeks, the colonel asked Paul's GP how long Paul was likely to be off work. During this conversation the GP told the colonel that Paul was an ex-drug addict (an unbeliev-able breach of patient confidentiality). The colonel sacked Paul immediately. Paul was devastated. A few days later he killed himself.

5

The common factor

The stress factor

In every condition encountered by the hypnotherapist there is one common factor; the common factor that is a component of every disease, every illness, every non-medical psychosomatic condition; a factor which can reduce the immune system's ability to combat bacterial and viral attack—stress.

An immune system in good health is capable of attacking and defeating just about every antigen. The natural killer cells B-cells, the detector T-cells; killer T-cells, lymphocytes, phagocytes, and macrophages are the parts of an army of defence which is stimulated into action by the ductless glands, the thymus and the hypothalamus. The hypothalamus is capable of producing hormones that trigger the production of norepinephrine, epinephrine, and corticosteroids, all of which are part of psychoneuroimmunology (PNI) and the greatest of these is psycho—the mind. Stress is a state of mind and is induced by fear and anxiety. Fear and anxiety stimulate another of the ductless glands, the pituitary, to release endorphins, a very powerful painkiller, into the bloodstream to help the system to cope with the fear or anxiety.

If an individual fails to cope, the state of mind becomes more stressful. The hypnotherapist's job is to initiate, in the first instance, changes in the state of mind in order to reduce the level of stress, thereafter using suggestion, and the client's imagination, to strengthen and stimulate the immune system in order to destroy the antigens that are invading the system.

The curse of the age?

To the lay person and to the medic alike the word 'stress' has a negative connotation. It is a condition with which we are all familiar, or at least we think we are. It is common practice to regard that which we call stress as the curse of our time. Yet how often do we hear a high achiever declare, 'I work better under pressure' or 'I work better to a deadline'? What they are really saying is 'I enjoy working under stress'. Outside of the working environment so many of us seek stress in our leisure pursuits. Mountain climbing, skiing, water skiing, competitive sailing, bungee jumping, sky diving, football, rugby, martial arts are all high-level stress activities, but what a high we get from the adrenalin rush!

Stress is often the motivating force that gets things done. We have negative and positive stresses. Some people experience both. There is the office worker or factory worker with a bad manager, who seeks positive stress at the weekend. What for one person may be a major disaster, for another may be a challenge to overcome. When the immediate situation or the environment impose demands on the person which exceed or are seen to exceed that person's ability to cope, then the sense of imbalance between the demand and capability constitutes a threat. Such a threat initiates physiological arousal that will activate the 'flight or fight' response. As the negative stress is ongoing and not resolved, the excess adrenalin will be damaging to the person's well-being. The emotional responses will also be psychologically damaging.

It is, of course, necessary to take into account, when dealing with long-standing problems, that the patient will in many cases have developed anxiety states associated with side issues that are inevitable in these situations; for example, in meetings, restaurants, theatres, cinemas, 'Where is the nearest lavatory?' 'How close is the nearest exit?' and 'How soon can I get out of here?' Even when these issues do not arise, there is the Free Floating Anxiety where the sufferer awakes every morning with a severe feeling of anxiety without any known source. It frequently happens that these two conditions exist without any single and independent instigator. A sufferer of inflammatory bowel syndrome (IBS) is frequently an anxious type and the two conditions may not be related and need quite different treatment. Apparently, gastrointestinal conditions are stress-related illnesses, so in this case it would be reasonable to assume that many gastrointestinal conditions may be responsive to hypnotherapy. It is acknowledged by the medical profession that 80 per cent of the symptoms presented to them during surgery hours are psychosomatic. After nearly twenty years in practice, I am convinced that there is no better treatment than hypnotherapy for such problems.

Mental or emotional

But these are physical solutions to physical issues. What about those other issues? Issues which do not involve invading antigens include: drug addiction, alcoholism, neurosis, anxiety, lack of confidence and low self-esteem, jealousy, frigidity, smoking, agoraphobia, claustrophobia, hysteria, and impotence. None of these are life threatening, although some might lead to life threatening situations, but every one of them not only seriously affects the quality of life of the sufferer, but also that of their extended family. Family life may be destroyed, and suicide is not uncommon. In cases of severe depression, the support and understanding that are so badly needed are frequently lacking, simply because family and close friends cannot understand what is happening to the sufferer, and how serious the situation is.

The common denominator is that these conditions are not created by antigen attack. There are no bacteria or viruses involved. These are not mental problems that can be regarded as a physical condition, but are emotional issues. Here we must differentiate between mental and emotional issues. Mental conditions are neurological, associated with the brain and the nervous system. Emotional diseases are psychosomatic in origin. They exist only in the mind. They do, of course, cause physical symptoms but, in the main, these symptoms disappear once the emotional issue is resolved. So how does the subconscious work its magic? People find it so easy to accept that the mind can cause disease but, strangely, they cannot accept that it can cure that which it has caused. Demonstrating that it does so, is only reiterating what is possible, not explaining how it is achieved. Can it all be the 'placebo effect' or is that a different and extra example of the magic of the subconscious?

The placebo effect

The placebo effect has frustrated and exasperated the medical and pharmaceutical professions for a hundred years. When 'double blind' tests are done to test the effectiveness of new treatments, the placebo groups invariably prove to be showing, on average, about 60 per cent as much benefit as the treatment. Indeed, in some cases it shows as great a benefit as a group receiving the drug or treatment being tested. One wonders how much of the placebo effect is responsible for the benefits gained by that group. If one considers this possibility, is it not possible that the placebo effect is even more effective than the test group? Will there come a time when we reject the use of drugs and depend instead on the healing power of the subconscious? Is such a thought so outrageous?

Suggestion in surgery

A television programme, screened in December 2002, showed a surgeon operating on a man who had a cartilage problem in his knee. For two years before the surgery, he had been in constant severe pain. Walking more than a few yards was virtually impossible, even with a stick.

Sylvester Colligan had the cartilage operation. Now after more than six years, he is still free from pain and walking freely. What he didn't know six years ago was that his operation was one of the placebo controls in a test that was designed to test the effectiveness of a variety of treatments. The results of the trial were reported in the Discovery Channel TV progamne called 'Placebo: Cracking the Code'.

The normal procedure is to open the knee surgically under general anaesthetic and smooth the torn cartilage by 'filing' the torn fibres and then closing the wound. In the case of Colligan, the surgeon opened the knee as usual but then simply closed the wound without doing any form of treatment. The result was amazing. Benefits for those patients who had the convential arthroscopy were no better than Colligan; he was told that the knee would now be perfectly sound. Checked six months later, the man was happily walking his dog without any difficulty and without a stick. He said the knee was fine. The placebo effect in surgery!

In an interview with the *Daily Telegraph*, Dr Alan Watkins, lecturer in medicine at the Southampton General Hospital, was reported as saying:

> *'There is now a substantial amount of evidence demonstrating that an individual's thoughts, feelings and spirit can have a profound effect on their endocrine, autonomic, cardio-respiratory, gastrointestinal and immune systems. A physician's attitude and approach can significantly influence a patient's mental, emotional and physical well-being,, either stimulating or handicapping recovery.'*

In the same article, Dr Michael Dixon, a Devon GP went even further:

> *'The placebo effect is the strongest, most comprehensive and most proven medicine available to GPs. A proper understanding of it could greatly improve our therapeutic effect and reduce the cost of medicine and procedures.'*

If this is possible, and demonstrably it is—and this is not an isolated case, it just happens to be one that was shown, in action, on television—then what is not possible?

There has been such progress in hypnotherapy during the past two decades that things which were thought to be impossible in the 1960s are now matter of course. David Elman, who was in his day the most famous hypnotist in America—he taught hypnotherapy to doctors and dentists (and only to doctors and dentists) between 1959 and 1977— stated in an interview with a doctor who was also his student , 'you can't stop a drinker from drinking, for life' and 'I have never heard of anyone being able to do so' (Elman, 1964: p323). I have in my filing cabinet letters from alcoholics thanking me for enabling them to stop drinking.

A fifteen-year success story

In the case of Stan (see p.78) it is, of now, fourteen years since he had a drink. He still turns up at my consulting room from time to time accompanied by his wife, two adult sons and a daughter who has her own children, and bringing along someone who needs help. In the voice of an ex-sergeant major, his first words to me as he stands to attention in the doorway of my consulting room are always the same. 'Haven't had a drink.' I am sure the reason he brings along his family is symbolic. When he first came to see me, his wife said, 'Alcoholism has destroyed our family. We don't have a family life anymore.' He wanted to demonstrate that this was no longer the case.

Premenstrual syndrome

The area of treatment that can give the greatest benefit to the largest group of people must surely be that scourge of most women—premenstrual syndrome (PMS), once better known as premenstrual tension (PMT). There is a mounting body of evidence to support the theory that stress is a major factor in the cause of this condition.

It has been frequently advocated that patients must practise self -ypnosis techniques over protracted periods in order to control this condition, but we consider this is an outdated practice. Such advances in methods and techniques have been made during the past twenty years that, in the author's experience, these stress-related conditions can often be resolved in three or four sessions of hypnotherapy using strong direct suggestion and post-hypnotic suggestion and, in some rare cases, the condition has been relieved in one session. However, a minimum of three sessions has always been given just to ensure that the benefits are lasting.

Cancer

The most frightening threat to health, dreaded above all others, must be the diagnosis of cancer. Department of Health statistics of 2000 state that one person in every three will develop cancer and one person in every four will die with it. That means there are about 16 million people suffering some form of cancer in the United Kingdom and in 2000 more than 270,000 people were diagnosed.

Hundreds of years before Christ, the most forward thinkers of their time recognised the relationship between mind and body. Hippocrates, who is recognised by historians as the 'father of medicine', believed 'Whatever happens in the mind influences the body.'

It is important to bear in mind the primary aim in the hypnotic induction, which is the ability to induce a state of very deep relaxation. During the past twenty years, evidence has shown a strong element of stress in the make-up of many cancer patients. Long-term suppression of anger, guilt and an inability to cope in stressful situations are frequent components of those prone to cancer (Eysenck, 1994). So it is reasonable to expect the hypnotic trance state to form the basis of a system of stress release that enhances the functioning of the immune system in the fight against cancer cells.

Hypnosis is an especially effective therapy for cancer sufferers who experience loss of self-esteem and confidence. Ego-strengthening suggestions enable patients to access the full potential of their own resources—by inducing a state of deep relaxation leading to hypnosis, then asking them to remember a time in the past when they felt really good about themselves. This could be a time when they achieved something that made them feel elated, not necessarily in a competitive situation but perhaps when their parents or a close companion said 'Well done'. Suggestions can then be given that this feeling will stay with them, each day growing better, stronger, more confident. 'Every day in every way getting better and better' (after Coué).

Not all members of the medical profession accept that the placebo effect or the power of suggestion is responsible for these healings. Healing often occurs spontaneously even when nothing is done to treat the illness or the injury. Many conditions and disorders fluctuate greatly, worsening or improving without apparent cause. It may be, they suggest, that the placebo is being given the credit for what is really a natural spontaneous healing—the body healing itself without outside intervention. However, people who are given no treatment very often do not do as well as those who are given placebos or convential treatment. A well-known factor in the healing process is just receiving medical care. The 'bedside manner' of old-fashioned family doctors often played a major role in a patient's recovery. An article by Margaret Talbot makes the point:

> *There is certainly data that suggests that just being in the healing situation accomplishes something. Depressed patients who are merely put on a waiting list for treatment do not do as well as those given a placebo. And this is very telling—when placebos are given for pain management, the course of pain relief follows what you would get with an active drug. The peak relief comes about an hour after it's administered, as it does with the real drug, and so on. If placebo analgesia was the equivalent of giving nothing, one would expect a more random pattern.'*

Margaret Talbot (2000)

6

Techniques

The first twenty minutes

Hypnotherapy and the placebo have a common denominator—suggestion. The mere act of being given the medicine in the medical environment—doctor's surgery, hospital, the white coat, stethoscope round the neck, instructions for taking the dosage—all reinforce the power of the suggestion 'this will make you better'. For hundreds of years, the patient's recovery depended more on their faith in the doctor or healer than on the treatments available.

Belief and faith

In the practice of hypnotherapy, the subject's faith in the practitioner and hypnotherapy is all important, far more important than the patient's faith in a doctor. Except in cases of paranoia or phobia, the patient is unlikely to be afraid of the doctor but many people fear hypnosis—it is the unknown. The hypnotherapist's first responsibility is to calm those anxieties; to make the unknown, known.

The misconceptions most people have about hypnosis must be dealt with first . We call this 'The First Twenty Minutes' and during this period we must still the anxieties that are the greatest obstacle to a successful outcome. But we never promise that 'This really will work'. One therapist was heard to say to his patient/client, 'I give you my personal guarantee that this will work for you.' That should never happen. It is to do with the 'Law of Reverse Effect'. If you say to someone, 'Do not think of a blue baboon', you know exactly what that person will do. They will have a mental picture of a blue monkey. The purpose of the first twenty minutes is to impart confidence in the ability of the subconscious mind to make those changes that are necessary in order to achieve the desired outcome. If you tell your patient/client, 'This really will be successful', they will start to think of failure.

Probably the most common misconception is that during hypnosis one is unconscious of what is happening and, on recovering full consciousness, will be without any memory of what has taken place. This is not true. It is important to explain that the subject is fully aware while in hypnosis and will hear everything and be able to remember everything. On a lighter note, it should be explained that we do not use any gadgets or gimmicks; no flashing lights, spinning discs, or swinging watches—we are simply taking advantage of the differences in the way the conscious and the subconscious minds work, that they have different capabilities and do different jobs. It is because of the differences that we are able to help people to make the changes they desire. The more information people have about the way these changes can be achieved, the more successful is the process. It is beneficial to explain the power of the subconscious mind to initiate change in emotional, mental and physical conditions and how, in hypnosis, we are able to bypass the conscious mind and talk directly to the subconscious, giving it instructions and suggestions that will initiate the desired changes. This is a very simplistic explanation of a very complex process but gives the patient/client an understanding of what is going on.

Having explained why hypnotherapy works so well, we then need to describe in detail just what is going to happen throughout the induction. It is important to do this because we need people to pay careful attention to what we are saying. The likelihood is that instead of giving us all their attention they will, at various stages of the induction, be wondering what is going to happen next. If we explain in advance exactly what is going to happen we have a better chance of keeping their attention.

A full explanation

For the purpose of this book I shall assume that the therapist is going to use a slightly modified version of the Elman technique (this technique will be explained in detail later). I consider this to be one of the most powerful, if not the most powerful, of all hypnosis techniques. For the 'Elman' we have the patient sitting in a very comfortable reclining chair with a foot rest: an Indian blanket of stiff cotton gives ladies a feeling of security, but is also used for men. The following is an introduction to the 'Elman', not the actual induction, but a description of the process:

> I shall start by asking you to look at that spot on the wall. I shall then ask you to open and close your eyes several times, each time you close your eyes I want you to still be focusing on that spot, as though you are looking through your eyelids. As you close your eyes, I want you to be thinking that you are allowing your eyelids to relax. After doing that several times I shall ask you to use your imagination. I want you to count backwards from 100. I want you to imagine you are looking at a blackboard, just as though you are back at school. On the blackboard will appear the number 100. When you see the number 100 you say it out loud. You then mentally wipe it away but as you wipe it away the next number appears and so on. Don't worry now, you will only have to count five or six numbers, we're not going all the way to zero. Having done that I shall ask you to imagine that you are standing in a lift—you don't have any problem with lifts, do you? I shall tell you the lift is going to go down through three levels—level A, level B and level C. I shall describe the interior of the lift to you and tell you that the lift will go down when I click my fingers. Having gone down through the three levels to level C, I shall say that I am going to count to three and tell you to open your eyes but when you do open your eyes you just keep them open till I click my fingers and say sleep and you close your eyes and allow yourself to drift off into a lovely sleepy state.

The Elman technique described above is one of the three techniques we use most frequently. Dave Elman was, in his day, the most famous hypnotist in America. He was a great teacher of hypnosis and taught only doctors and dentists. He considered his techniques too powerful for lay people. He was born on 6 May 1900 in North Dakota and died on 5 December 1965. The Elman technique we teach our students is a slightly modified version based on the tapes made in his own voice during his teaching course.

There are many induction techniques and every professional hypnotherapist has his/her own favourite inductions. For the purpose of this book we refer only to techniques we have used on a daily basis over the past twenty years.

The Physical Relaxation Induction

The Elman technique requires the use of visualisation and occasionally we meet a person who has great difficulty in visualising—some find it impossible. The use of the lemon test quickly identifies these people (see Chapter 4, p.65). In these cases, we use a physical relaxation which is ideal for use in group situations and is similar to relaxation techniques used in many other disciplines; but the start of the relaxation begins with the following instruction:

> I am going to start with your feet. I shall first tell you to think of your feet and then after a few seconds I shall tell you to think of your feet relaxing. Now, this is important; when I tell you to think of your feet I don't want you to dwell upon that thought, I just want you to let the thought pass through your mind without paying it any attention. When, a few seconds later I tell you to think of your feet relaxing, I want you to treat that thought in just the same way as the first one. Don't dwell upon it, don't concentrate on it, above all don't TRY to relax your feet. Just let that thought pass through your mind as did the first thought. I shall then continue to do the same thing with all the parts of your body, first of all identifying the part, for example the muscles of your shins, and then telling you to think of them relaxing and every time you do it just as you did with the thoughts of your feet.

This may seem like a very long-winded introduction to a simple relaxation technique, but it is very effective and can be used just as successfully with a roomful of people as in a one-to-one situation. The subject is so involved in following the instructions that the relaxation occurs almost subliminally.

Music a powerful adjunct

During this technique we always use music. Select a soothing piece of music, played very quietly in the background. Ideally the selection should be a short phrase without much change in volume, i.e. about three or four minutes long, and making a continuous loop. Apart from the fact that the music aids relaxation, it also serves a secondary purpose—if any extraneous noise occurs during the relaxation process, a disturbing effect is very much reduced if it does not fall into a total silence.

Having completed the physical relaxation, we proceed with a process to relax the mind, saying to our subject:

> I am now going to count from one to fifteen. Between each number I count, I shall be talking to you about relaxation. By the time we reach fifteen, you will be deeply relaxed both in body and mind. I shall count to three and on the count of three I shall tell you to open your eyes. When you do open your eyes you keep them open until I click my fingers and say 'Sleep now' when you close your eyes and go deep into the sleep state we call hypnosis.

The suggestions used during this counting should be related to the issue to be resolved. The following is an example of a general relaxation technique.

> **One**: You are feeling warm and comfortable pleasantly relaxed.
>
> **Two**: Be aware only of the beautifully relaxing music and the sound of my voice.
>
> **Three**: Listening to my voice, you feel soothed, relaxed, secure.
>
> **Four**: You feel so relaxed. Such a beautiful feeling.
>
> **Five**: As though you are floating away on a great calm smooth ocean of tranquillity.

Six: Floating away beneath lovely blue sky. Watching little white clouds floating slowly across that lovely blue sky.

Seven: And as each little white cloud drifts so slowly across the lovely blue sky you feel yourself relaxing even deeper.

Eight: Drifting with the music, listening to my voice. Relaxing deeper ever deeper.

Nine: Just let go and drift away. Feeling so sleepy now.

Ten: Feeling so happy. So secure. A wonderful, wonderful feeling.

Eleven: Nothing shall disturb you now. Drifting into deeper ever deeper levels of relaxation.

Twelve: No longer awake nor yet asleep. In a never, never land somewhere between the two.

Thirteen: Drifting with the music listening to my voice. So soothing so relaxing. Going deeper, ever deeper.

Fourteen: And when I count fifteen all you want to do is to let go completely and drift away into this lovely sleep state.

Fifteen: So tired now . So drowsy. So sleepy now. In a moment I shall count to three; on the count of three I shall tell you to open your eyes. When you do open your eyes you keep them open till I click my fingers and say 'Sleep now' when you close your eyes and go deep asleep.

Magic of subconscious

We hypothesise that it is the power of suggestion via the subconscious mind that initiates the required change. It is important to bear in mind that the behavioural outcomes achieved through hypnotherapy are, to a very significant extent, subliminal. For example:

> Simon was middle-aged of medium height, dark hair and very pale features. He was breathing heavily after climbing a flight of twenty stairs. His doctor had told him that he must stop smoking. He was suffering from emphysema. Stopping smoking could considerably extend his life expectancy (for the stop smoking programme we have a two sessions within a five-day period). The first session

took him easily into deep hypnosis. His was judged to be a case for strong direct suggestion. The therapy proceeded as follows:

'Now Simon, your subconscious mind is fully aware of your need to overcome the smoking habit and because it is your will, because it is your sincere desire and your very urgent need, your subconscious mind will bring about those changes in your behaviour which will ensure that from the time that I tell you to wake up again today you are a non-smoker for the rest of your life.

You will experience no side effects.

You will experience no ill effects.

It will be as though you have never been a smoker.

There will be no cravings. You feel no desire for cigarettes. You feel no need to smoke. Your body is free of the smoking habit. Your bloodstream is free of the nicotine addiction. You are a non-smoker for the rest of your life. The thought does not enter your mind.

Even though people around you are smoking it will not trouble you in any way at all. Even though the room you are in is full of cigarette smoke that will not bother you in any way.

There will be no side effects of any kind. You will feel no need to eat extra food of any kind to compensate for not smoking, it will be as though you have never been a smoker. You are a non-smoker for the rest of your life and you feel good about that. You are happy with that. You congratulate yourself. You have beaten your smoking habit and you feel good about yourself.

All these suggestions are reiterated two or three times changing the wording slightly each time.

Attending for his second session he reported that he had not smoked and that he hadn't even thought about smoking; in fact, it had been many hours before he realised that he hadn't smoked. The behavioural changes had taken place subliminally. This type of direct suggestion is very powerful and strongly recommended wherever the circumstances seem appropriate and may be used, suitably modified, to deal with many different issues. This is an example of just one of hundreds of 'stop smoking' sessions.

The healing mind

Hypnotherapy's greatest benefit must be to be able to heal oneself. The power of the human subconscious to self heal has been demonstrated over and again by the placebo effect.

Many years ago I awoke one morning to find that I had a stiff neck. It was very painful. I fully expected it to get better within a day or two but it didn't get better, it got worse. Eventually I went to a doctor who sent me to a hospital. After tests and X-rays I was told that I had a condition called Cervical Spondulosis, that there was no cure and that it would get worse. I attended the Leeds General Hospital three times a week over a period of three years as an out-patient, receiving all sorts of treatments: infra-red, ultra-violet, traction, etc., in an attempt to alleviate the pain. Nothing worked. It became so painful that the slightest movement of my head was agony. At the time I had a very responsible job which involved a lot of driving. I had to take along a passenger whose job was to look sideways for me because I could not turn my head. One day, driving home, I pulled into a lay-by.

'It's no good' I said to my passenger 'I just can't go on without a rest. My neck is so painful.'

My passenger, a young lady who was an old friend of my family, and who had often heard me speak of my belief in the power of the body to heal itself turned in her seat and said 'If you really believe all you say about the power of the mind to heal, why don't you heal yourself?'

I was really shaken. I had suffered this awful pain for nearly three years and never once given a thought to the possibility of healing myself. The doctors had told me that it was incurable and I had believed them.

Without replying to her I sat back in my seat and went into deep relaxation. I repeated to myself over and over 'I shall be free from pain for ten minutes.' I kept saying that until at last I felt the pain receding. I was able to drive home free from pain for the first time for three years. The next morning the first thing I did was to repeat the same process, but this time I specified twenty minutes free from pain. It worked again. I did it every morning, gradually extending the time. Three weeks later I was completely free from pain. But there was an amazing bonus. Not only was I free from pain but it seemed that the condition which was said to be incurable was completely cured. It has never returned and that was over 30 years ago.

How is that possible?

I don't know. Having worked and studied in the field for over twenty years, I am still like the man who switched on his electric light 70 years ago. I know what to do to make it work but how it works is still a mystery. In spite of all that fascinating information emanating from the psychological, neurological and psychiatric laboratories telling us exactly what happens in the brain when stimulation is applied under hypnosis, we still do not know how the human mind does what it does to bring about those changes, which are not only emotional, and mental but—as in the case of the cartilage surgery—also physical.

It is true that during the past 25 to 30 years there has been considerable research into the neuropsychophysiology of hypnosis, especially in America and Australia, and we now have considerably more information about the physical and chemical changes in different loci of the brain observed under various test conditions. This is very interesting to the academic but of little help to the therapist. It tells us what is happening and where it is happening in the brain but it does not tell us how that activity brings about behavioural change in the patient.

In her book *Neuropsychophysiology of Hypnosis: Towards an Understanding of How Hypnotic Interventions Work*, Helen J Crawford writes:

> 'During the transition from the 1900s, labelled the "Decade of the Brain", into the twenty-first century, new discoveries about the neuropyschophysiological bases of hypnosis are being made. The excitement is high as interdisciplinary approaches address old and new questions about psychological and physiological

phenomena with ever-refined electro-physiological neuroimaging techniques. Hypnosis and its various phenomena should have neuropyschophysiological correlates if one takes to heart a quote from Miller, Galanter and Pribram's (1960) seminal book "Plans and the Structure of Behaviour": "There is good evidence for the age old belief that the brain has something to do with—Mind."'

Crawford and Gruzelier (1992: p.196)

Brainwaves

The brain functions on four different vibrations:
Alpha = 8hz to15hz
Beta = 14hz to 30hz
Theta = 4hz to 8hz
Delta = up to 4hz

Eyes wide open, alert and fully aware of your environment, you're in beta; depending on your level of attention, somewhere between 14 to 30 Hertz. Eyes closed, not thinking of anything in particular, you're in alpha, somewhere between 8 to 15 Hertz. Sitting in the sun, eyes closed, drifting into a day-dream, or in hypnosis, you're in theta, somewhere between 4 to 8 Hertz. Sound asleep and probably dreaming or maybe in a coma, you're in delta, somewhere below 4 Hertz. One Hertz equals one beat per second.

The theta state can only exist in the brain when there is a complete absence of stress in the mind. The vast majority of us grow up in a stable family background where we absorb the knowledge of right and wrong from our parents' teaching and from their example. By the time we are four or five years old, we have become conditioned to accept the 'rules' of the society in which we live. That conditioning affects all our behaviour for the rest of our lives. Even if later in life we were to break all the laws of society, that early conditioning would still affect us.

If we contemplate doing something which we have been conditioned to believe is wrong, a state of stress will exist in our mind. That condition of stress will prevent us achieving the theta state and the wrong which we are contemplating will create stress within our own mind.

It is impossible to contemplate something which is against one's own moral code when in a theta state. Such thoughts would break the state because of the stress it introduces. The theta state is a trance state. Whether induced by a hypnotherapist or achieved by practising meditative techniques, it makes little difference. Just in case you are thinking that there are people who do not have a very high moral code, I am of the opinion that such people are unlikely to be interested in theta states.

Self-healing and theta

For some people the greatest benefit to be gained from achieving theta would be self-healing. That was probably an understatement. The ability to heal one's self is such an asset that there is unlikely to be anybody who is not interested to some extent. Even if not suffering from any illness at this time, we are all liable to suffer injuries or illness.

The human mind is capable of healing both body and mind of almost any ailment or injury which may afflict us. That may seem a very rash statement, but it is true. The trained human mind is able to control every aspect of the body's functioning. It can alter the heart beat, increase or reduce the metabolic rate, reduce the body's demand for oxygen, raise or lower body temperature, render any part of the body immune to pain, or stimulate the immune system to fight off attacks by bacteria or viruses. In fact, until quite recently, the main reason people recovered from an illness was because the body healed itself. The remedies the medical profession provided were worse than useless. People got better in spite of the doctor's treatment, not because of it.

Ignorance not incompetence

This was not really the fault of the medical profession. They genuinely believed that their treatments were beneficial, but the most effective medicine they had was their own belief in their prescriptions. They told the patient that this or that medicine would cure them. Because the patient had faith in the doctor and the doctor believed in his medicine, the patient frequently recovered.

It is difficult for us in this more enlightened age to understand, for example, how the doctors of the day could believe that a patient, weakened by illness, could benefit from bloodletting. Yet they frequently took as much as half a pint of blood from a seriously ill patient in the belief that it would cure a fever.

Emile Coué's Laws of Suggestion

About a hundred years ago, a French chemist, Emile Coué, discovered quite by accident just how powerful was the human mind's ability to heal its own body. In Coue's day the chemist had to make up the prescriptions himself. There were no major drug companies to supply him with ready-made medicines. Whatever the doctor prescribed, the chemist had to formulate from his own stock of chemicals.

Coué's shop was a busy one and he kept a stock of the most commonly used prescriptions already made up. He was busy making up stock prescriptions one day when into his shop came a customer he knew only too well. This was a man who had been ill for many months. Almost every week he came to Coué and complained that the medicine Coué had given him last week had done him no good.

On this particular day Coué was feeling harassed. There had been lots of customers in the shop and he had some difficult prescriptions to make up. As he listened to this customer's complaints Coué became more and more irritated. At last he reach up to a shelf above his head, took a bottle of pale pink liquid and slammed it down on his counter with such a bang that the bottle was in danger of breaking.

'Take this,' he exclaimed, 'it is the very latest from Paris. You'll be better within the week.'

The man was considerably shaken by Coué's attitude and scuttled from the shop without another word. A week later that same man was back. Coué, fed up of the sight of the man, was about to order him out of the shop when the customer dashed forward. Grabbing Coué by the hand he cried, 'Thank you, thank you. That medicine you gave me last week was wonderful. I'm completely cured.'

Coué was astonished. The bottle had contained nothing more than coloured water with a little flavouring. It had no medicinal content at all. It was a stock mixture to which he would have added whatever medicine was required. For a long time Coué pondered about that bottle of coloured water.

He eventually decided that the man had been cured because he had believed what Coué had told him, in other words he was cured by his own belief. The man had cured himself. From this one experience Coué developed a whole system of healing by suggestion, which became very popular in the early 1920s, especially in America, and was known as Couéism. His followers were taught to assert daily 'Every day in every way I am better and better'. Coué also developed what he called the three laws of suggestion.

(1) If logic and emotion are in accord it is not as if they are added together but as though they are multiplied by each other;

(2) If logic and emotion are in opposition, emotion will always win;

(3) Logic is unchangeable. Emotion can be changed.

That last is probably the most important.

Self-healing and suggestion

Healing by suggestion is really self-healing, and it is something mankind has been doing for thousands of years. Ever since the days when we lived in caves and dressed in animal skins, there have been those who practised as healers. They used all sorts of rituals and so-called magic potions, but all the rituals did was to reinforce the suggestion that if those rituals were carried out then you would get well again. They were very effective. Is that very different from the mother who picks up a hurt child and says, 'Never mind darling, let mummy kiss it better and all the hurt will go away'?

How does this, seemingly miraculous, healing work and why? The aspect of the mind called the subconscious has recorded within itself everything there is to know about the body and the mind. It knows everything there is to know about you and everything which has ever happened to you. It knows the state of health of every cell of your being. If any part of you is out of harmony, your subconscious knows about it and is capable of doing whatever is necessary to restore the balance and make you well again. But in order to do that, it is essential for your body and mind to be in a state of complete rest—in deep relaxation.

The immune system in relaxation

In our modern world we live in such a state of stress that the subconscious is never given the opportunity to heal. The human brain is capable of producing within itself—or instructing other glands of the body to produce—any of the chemicals needed to restore the body to health. The white cells in our bloodstream are responsible for attacking and destroying bacteria or viruses which invade our bodies and the only way we can recover from a virus infection is by defeating it with our own immune system.

So you see, not only is self-healing possible, without it you would die young. One of its uses is in the control of pain. If you hurt yourself, for example on your hand, grasp your wrist with the other hand and as you go into instant relaxation you say to yourself very firmly, 'The pain response will not go beyond my wrist. It will not reach my brain. I shall feel no pain.'

Here is another tip; if you should happen to scald yourself or burn yourself, then add to the declaration, the words 'It will not blister, I shall feel no pain.' You will, of course, modify the message to fit the injury, and, using your common sense, go to the cold tap and run cold water over the burn. Don't ever forget common sense.

Do you suffer with frequent headaches? Try this. Sit in relaxation. Focus your attention in the very centre of the headache. Now move the pain two inches to one side. Stay in the centre of the pain. Now move it to the other side. Still keep in the centre of the pain. Now move it two inches backward. Stay in the centre of the pain. Now move it two inches *above* your head. *It has gone*.

A word about headaches. Many people who suffer from frequent headaches are people who get stressed. The headache is caused by tension in the muscles of the upper back, between the shoulder blades. That requires massage of those muscles and the muscles of the back of the neck and the scalp to get rid of the headache properly. Otherwise the pain will return.

The technique of self-healing is the same no matter what the problem. You do not name the condition. You have gone into this ASC for the express purpose of treating your condition. You don't need to mention it by name. Tell yourself, 'My mind and my body shall act in harmony to cure me of this condition.'

Do this every day, repeat the message ten times each time you do it. Don't say 'I *want* my mind and my body to act—etc,' you must say, 'My mind and my body *shall* act together to cure me of this condition.'

Phobias defeated

There are many, many people whose quality of life is ruined by a phobia. Phobias can vary from being a minor nuisance to being a source of major panic states which induce feelings of sheer terror.

The following technique has proved very powerful in curing phobias, anxiety and fears of many kinds. Having taken the subject into hypnosis, the following suggestions are given:

Imagine you are sitting in a cinema; you are alone in the cinema. The screen lights up as the projectionist starts the film rolling. You see a picture of yourself on the screen.

The picture is in full colour. You see that picture of yourself standing on the left side of the screen and in the centre of the screen is the situation of which you are afraid. You realise that you are seeing this from a different perspective. You are no longer in the auditorium, you are in the projection box. Looking down from the projection box, you can see yourself sitting in auditorium watching the screen. You are twice removed from what is happening on the screen. You feel very relaxed as you watched that self on the screen walk towards the centre of the screen.

Sitting in your cinema seat you are far removed from that image on the screen so you feel quite relaxed and at ease.

The you on the screen must walk right into the centre of the phobic situation and just as the you on the screen reaches the very centre of the phobic situation the picture switches from full colour to black and white and instantly the picture starts to run backwards very fast. You know what it looks like when a cine picture runs in reverse. It looks funny doesn't it?

It runs in reverse right back to the beginning again. And then it turns back to full colour and starts again. Repeat that process three times. Do that every day for a week and you will get rid of your phobia.

I know it sounds very complicated and a lot to remember, but read this several times and get the sequence fixed in your mind. It really isn't as difficult as it seems. There is just one thing I must add. There are some people who are unable to see a visualisation in colour no matter how they try. If you are one of these people, it is just something you have to accept. For you the pictures may always be in black and white. Some people always dream in black and white. It is just one of those things. Don't let it put you off. The visualisations will be just as effective in black and white.

Agoraphobia

'Agoraphobia'—loosely translated from the Greek as fear of the market place—has, over recent years, acquired a wider meaning than when it was originally introduced although it is still so used in some countries. In Britain it is now taken to include fears not only of open spaces, but also of related aspects, such as the presence of crowds and the difficulty of immediate easy escape to a safe place, quite often the sufferer's car, but usually the home. It is not uncommon for the agoraphobic to be unable to leave his/her own home. This label often refers to an interrelated and overlapping cluster of phobias embracing fears of leaving home, of entering shops, crowds, and public places, or of travelling in public transport. Although the severity of the anxiety and the extent of avoidance behaviour vary considerably, this is the most incapacitating of the phobic disorders and many sufferers become completely housebound, terrified by the thought of collapsing and being left helpless in public. The lack of an immediately available exit is one of the key features of many of these agoraphobic situations. Most sufferers are women and the onset is usually early in adult life but re-active agoraphobia can occur at any stage of life. Depressive and obsessional symptoms and social phobias may also be present but do not dominate the clinical picture. In the absence of effective treatment, agoraphobia becomes chronic, and invariably gets worse.

Secondary benefits

It is as well to bear in mind that some agoraphobics experience little anxiety because they create for themselves a compatible environment. The presence of sympathetic family members or close friends who accept that the agoraphobic is incapable of self-help and act as 'carers', doing the shopping, taking the sufferer for drives in the car (many agoraphobics are able to go for a drive in a car but unable to get out of the car at the destination), and fetching and carrying outside the home. The agoraphobic may adapt to this situation so completely that there is resistance to change. To one who has been agoraphobic for many years, change may mean taking responsibility for many aspects of one's life that have been taken care of by others. The presence or absence of anxiety in the agoraphobic situation may be an indication of the existence of a secondary benefit.

Mishap on the motorway

Simon was the last sort of man to have a disabling phobia—a big strong looking fellow, who worked out in the gym two or three times a week. In his early 40s, he had risen through the ranks. From being a sales representative he was now the general sales manager of an international company with many area sales managers and an army of salesmen on the road. Like so many successful business men, he lived in a pleasant rural area an hour's drive from his office in the city. On this day he was half an hour from the office when the traffic slowed to a halt on the motorway. This was not an uncommon state of affairs and Simon sat, quite relaxed reflecting on the day ahead, fully expecting to be on the move again in a few minutes. What Simon didn't know was that the hold-up was caused by a major accident involving dozens of vehicles. He gradually became aware of discomfort in his tummy. He needed a lavatory. He was in the outside lane. In front and behind the traffic was solid as far as could be seen. The situation got worse. Eventually he could control it no longer. He was in a horrible mess physically as well as emotionally. By a fortunate coincidence his wife was already in the city having caught an early train in order to meet a friend. They both had mobile phones. How he got out of that mess and into his office in a clean suit is a long story and not relevant to this book.

A few days later he decided he would leave home a little early in order to use the A-road instead of the motorway, just in case. A couple of days later he was due to go to the airport to meet some foreign buyers. He felt that he couldn't risk having these passengers in his car, just in case. He sent his PA. Within a very short while, he was making excuses for not taking anyone anywhere in his car. He was travelling to his office by train, pretending that the car was in need of repair after a minor accident. He told no one of his problem, not even his wife. He was becoming desperate, conscious of the fact that if he did not overcome the problem his career was in danger.

The situation came to a head when one evening his wife told Simon that their two daughters wished to spend part of the summer vacation touring inland France, away from the tourist places, in order to meet the people and to practise their French. The vacation was only weeks away. He had to tell his wife of his problem. She suggested he try hypnotherapy.

I knew as soon as we met that Simon was a strong, positive confident man in every respect except this one and I decided that strong direct suggestion, plus powerful post-hypnotic suggestion, would be the best way to deal with the issue. Using the physical relaxation induction with deepening suggestions, I gave him positive suggestions that he would be completely at ease with passengers in his car no matter who they were and that from the moment he approached his car he would be relaxed and at ease and able to enjoy the journey no matter who was in the car with him; whether on motorways or minor roads, it made no difference at all. These and similar suggestions were given over a series of four sessions. I next heard of Simon about three months later when he phoned me to say that he had recently enjoyed a long tour of France with his family that had been a great success.

7

The child in healthcare

People frequently doubt the ability of children to respond adequately to hypnosis but there is plenty of historical evidence to the contrary. Since the Franklin Commission of 1748 concluded, in their investigation into Mesmer, that the documented clinical benefits were not due to magnetism but were in their view due to the patient's imagination, one can easily understand that children, with their vivid imaginations, would make excellent subjects for healing based on suggestion.

Before the days when chemical anaesthetics became available, both Braid and Elliotson were able to successfully induce hypnotic anaesthesia in child patients to alleviate their suffering during surgery.

Early reports

An English hypnotherapist, J Milne Bramwell, in his textbook of 1903, and two French doctors, Liebault and Bernheim, all reported the use of hypnosis with problems such as bed-wetting, nail biting and recurring headaches. But the USA lagged behind in this application of therapy and little progress was made until the late 1950s and 1960s, when Drs Milton Erickson and Erik Wright reported their successful use of child hypnosis and the paediatrician Dr Franz Bauman's skill in treating children in hypnosis made him the first paediatrician to become the President of the American Society of Clinical Hypnosis.

The ability of most children to drift easily between fantasy and reality makes them good subjects for hypnotic intervention in many areas of child healthcare. Benefit has been reported in cases of chronic illnesses, such as cancer, haemophilia and asthma (Olness and Kohen, 1996). The training of children in the use of self-hypnosis techniques has been particularly successful but it is of prime importance for the practitioner to study carefully the child's mental development. A ten-year-old may have the mental age of seven or twelve years, so using the appropriate language to suit the child's mental age is often the key to gaining their attention.

Guided imagery and visualisation

The natural spontaneous shifts into altered states are accompanied by visualisations which may be employed to heighten suggestibility and focus attention. While it is difficult, and sometimes impossible, for a child of six or seven years to relax to the level which would be induced in adult hypnosis, it is not necessary and should not be expected as a norm. Experience indicates that a child of twelve years and upwards is in the majority of cases sufficiently literate to be able to understand and co-operate as well as adults, and enjoy even better levels of success providing that the introductory 'first twenty minutes' is suitably edited to ensure a full understanding of terms such as the subconscious mind. The use of guided imagery or visualisation is of prime importance and is found to be a powerful tool in cases of enuresis, nail biting, thumb sucking, hair pulling and self-harm.

Pain

Children in acute pain are often the easiest patients to help with the use of hypnotic techniques because they are highly motivated to feel better, to re-establish a sense of control in their life, and to rid themselves of pain, or at least decrease their discomfort. In an office, emergency room, urgent care centre, or even at an accident site, it is important to speak to an injured or ill child in a manner at once reassuring, comforting and believable. Children in an emergency situation of acute pain are already in a spontaneous, negatively focused, hypnotic state, negative in its acutely focused concentration on the injury, the bleeding, and the fear that things will get worse (Kohen, 1986; Kuttner, 1997; Olness and Kohen, 1996). It is, therefore, that much more important to choose our language of communication carefully, and modulate what we say and how we say it to foster attention toward positive feelings, expectations, and ultimately co-operation. When a clinician empathically tells an emergency room child-patient, 'Whew... that really hurts', this immediately identifies the clinician as a good observer, fosters the child's willingness and ability to pay attention to the clinician, and opens the opportunity for additional hypnotic suggestions toward relief; for example, 'I'm glad you came to the doctor, it will probably hurt less soon' or 'It will probably keep right on hurting until it doesn't need to anymore...now that you're here—and know you will be getting help...'

Reframing techniques

Positive reframing expectations might easily be reinforced by hypnotic strategies designed to allow the child to alter his/her perception of discomfort; for example, we might say 'Would it be okay to take your mind somewhere else'?' or 'What will you do when you get home, after this is taken care of?' Beyond distraction, this query offers the reassurance to the child that she will be going home. Similarly, children in acute pain often accept direct 'permission' or suggestions to dissociate their pain; for example, 'Close your eyes. . . find the switches in your mind that control discomfort... Find the one for your leg... What colour is it in your mind'?... What shape? Is it a turn or a flip or a slide kind of switch? Now, turn it down... and then 1-2-3-click, off, and notice how different it feels... nice going!' Adding relaxation, dissociation via leaving to a favourite place, or hypnoanesthesia or analgesia by cleaning the injured part with a 'special liquid that is cool and comforting' are additional strategies that may be useful, especially as they are tailored to the child's needs (Kohen and Olness, 1993; Olness and Kohen, 1996).

For procedures such as injections, venipunctures for blood withdrawal or intra-venous hookups, a bone marrow or spinal tap, more time is usually available to plan treatment and hypnotic assistance. This allows for, and should include, a creative exploration of the techniques that may be of greatest benefit to a given child, and for rehearsal in preparation for the designated procedure. The use of hypnotically-induced amnesia of the pain of previous treatments is valuable in cases of repetitive procedures.

Chronic disease, terminal illness

In *No Fears, No Tears* and its sequel, *No Fears, No Tears—13 Years Later* (Kuttner, 1986; 1999), children with cancer demonstrate the range and usefulness of hypnotic techniques in helping themselves to modify discomfort, effectively manage difficult and repetitive medical procedures, and manage the effects of these challenging treatments. The use of guided visual imagery is one of the most effective ways of teaching children to control pain. A child who is suffering chronic pain can be taught the following visualisation and supplied with a tape to use daily or as needed; they will feel in control and able to help themself. The child is asked to imagine a place in which they would feel absolutely safe and comfortable, perhaps a place they know from previous experience, or perhaps a place they create in their imagination

Safe place induction

> **Safe place imagery**: Separate your hands and feet and put your back into a comfortable position that it can stay in for a long period of time. Close your eyes and allow yourself to imagine a safe place in nature where you've been before or plan to be, or you may just create it within yourself. Brighten up the colour and notice how clear it is and how good it feels to be there. Notice the things that are moving about and how clear and wonderful the mood is and free from discomfort. There may be a special scent in the air, a few clouds drifting gently across the sky—a sky that goes on forever and forever, a bright light that reaches you shining down between the clouds allowing you to feel warm, comfortable and relaxed. This light stands

for everything that's good in life, such as love, serenity, tranquillity, pure relaxation and perfect peace.

Allow this light to flow through the whole of your body from top to toe relaxing every muscle fibre, cell and tissue. As it flows through you from head to toe, allow it to completely relax each muscle group. As it begins to flow through the forehead, feel the discomfort simply melt away. It automatically continues to flow through the eyes as the thread muscles behind the eyes simply unravel and the eyes get heavier. The white light automatically continues to flow down over the temples and through the front of the neck...at the same time down the back of the head, neck and shoulders. Allow gravity to pull the shoulders down into their natural positions. The mind may wander and drift, or it may become drowsy and foggy. Whatever happens is completely natural; you'll still hear the relaxing sound of my voice, which is soon to become a comfortable feeling in the background. My words will soon blend into one another and flow into your mind naturally, so you'll be free from having to listen to the words as the subconscious will recognise what they mean anyway. And the mind simply unwinds like a big spring, letting go. This is just pure, simple relaxation. All fears, guilts and self-blame are released.

Plus breathing

Allow the white light to continue to flow through the elbows, wrists, and out the fingers. You may notice a tingling sensation within the hands, which further shows you are beginning to relax as the bodily functions are slowing down. The breathing becomes a shade deeper; with each more relaxing breath, feel the body rest more firmly against the pads that you're laying or sitting against.

As the white light flows down through the back, all the muscles and tendons wrapped around the vertebrae unwind and the back settles into its natural position automatically. The light flows through the waist, knees, ankles, and out through the toes. All stress, concerns, worries, in the form of tension or tightness, which may have been locked up in the body, are useless to us now. Feel the nerves dimming like dimming the lights.

And with each beat of the heart you are naturally more in touch, becoming relaxed in this way. Allow yourself to go deeper and deeper. The deeper you go the better you feel. You don't feel a thing now. Just a lovely relaxed happy feeling and that feeling will stay with you, every day in every way you feel better.

Studies indicate that children are able to use hypnotic skills to reduce nausea and vomiting (LaClave and Blix, 1989). With terminally ill children, hypnosis has been a particularly effective adjunctive modality in assisting them and their families to cope with and navigate those last moments (Gardner, 1976; Olness and Kohen, 1996). Many different images may be introduced into the guided visualisation. Creative visualisations involving fantasy situations such as 'flying up and away from the earth to float amongst the stars', and 'looking down on the earth like a great big jewel' are particularly effective.

In the case of very young children—five/six years old—a more down to earth relaxation has proved successful: 'Imagine you are going to the beach but there is a very big hill of sand between you and the beach. You have to climb that sandy hill and the sand is very soft. As you climb your feet sink into the sand. The sun is warm and you get so tired climbing up that sand. Just lie down and rest now.'

Anxiety

A sensitive, complete history and assessment, together with careful pacing of the emerging therapeutic relationship, will commonly yield ideas about the proper role of hypnotherapy for a particular child. For the common performance anxiety of stage fright, or palpitations or 'butterflies in the stomach' before a big game or a recital, it is often easily demonstrated to the child that his/her response, like a habit, has become a conditioned reaction association with negative expectations, and he/she can learn how it can be modified and mastered.

This may be accomplished easily by discussing the everyday phenomena of physiologic responses to stressful events. One easily understood example is that of blushing with embarrassment. The clinician can explain that one first experiences something, followed by feeling a reaction of embarrassment, followed—often instantaneously—by a physical response of blushing which in itself may be embarrassing. When the clinician asks the child if they stay blushed, they usually comment that they can and do act in some way to relieve the feeling of embarrassment, thus curtailing the blushing episode. This brief conversation can provide an everyday example of how a shift in the way a child *feels* can provide a shift in the physical response (of blushing) without even thinking about it. Graphic representation of changes in autonomic responsivity in response to feeling or 'thinking' changes can be even more dramatically demonstrated to children through computerised biofeedback reflection of EMG (electromyographic), EDA (electrodermal activity), or peripheral temperature changes during hypnosis, relaxation and imagery experiences (Culbert *et al*, 1994).

Guided visualisation

Guided visualisation has been found to be the approach of first choice by using the 'Frame Technique' (Morton Healey and Jean Murton, 1986), in which the child, in hypnosis, imagines himself looking at a large picture frame; in the picture frame is a blank canvas. The canvas may be any colour. In the centre of the frame the child sees an image of him/herself as he/she sees him/herself in present time: anxious, low self-esteem, lacking confidence, unhappy or whatever the problem may be. The child is then told to see another image of him/herself. This image appears on the extreme left side of the picture and it is an image of him/herself looking healthy, successful, happy, confident and relaxed, easily and confidently doing all those things that have been difficult or impossible in the past. That image of the new you then moves quickly into the centre of the picture and with great energy and strong purpose kicks the old you out of the picture; the new person is seen in the centre of the picture looking great and representing the him/her as being the person that he/she really wants to be, feeling relaxed and happy and feeling really good about him/herself. This process is then completed by the practitioner giving the post-hypnotic suggestion, 'From the moment that I tell you to wake up today, every hour of every day you become closer and closer to being the person that you really want to be.'

> *The use of hypnotherapy is often very effective in helping children and families with the common experience of separation anxiety: helping children with the natural but difficult process of grief and bereavement following the death of a grandparent or other relative. The use of positive imagery of happy memories, re-experienced by way of age regression, is very effective in this situation.'*

Olness and Kohen (1996)

Eating disorders

One of the most disturbing phenomena of our time is that of the obese child, in the majority of cases the obese girl child. Schachter (1971) reports that overweight people also seem to pay little attention to internal cues (e.g. hunger pangs) and base their eating habits more on external cues (e.g. the availability and taste of food). However, although there is some evidence that hypothalamic tumours are associated with obesity in obese humans, there is no evidence that the hypothalamus does not function properly in overweight people generally, although it is still possible that it works differently in 'fat' and 'thin' eaters.

Availability and apathy

Schachter *et al* (1968) found that while normal weight people responded to the internal cue of stomach distension ('feeling bloated') by refusing any more food, obese people tended to go on eating. Similarly, when a group of normal and a group of obese people were deprived of one meal and then half of each group was given a roast beef sandwich and the other half left hungry, only the normal weight people who had eaten the sandwich ate fewer crackers when allowed to eat their fill—the fact that some of the obese people had eaten a sandwich made no difference to the number of crackers they ate.

Schachter (1971) suggests that it is the availability of food to which the obese people were responding. However, he also found that they are less prepared than normal weight people to make an effort to find food (e.g. go into the next room to get sandwiches) or to prepare the food in some way (e.g. shell peanuts) so the former tend to keep on eating as long as food is in sight or is ready to eat, regardless of whether their physiological needs have been met, while the latter are more willing to search for food but only if they are genuinely hungry.

Overweight people also tend to report that they feel hungry at prescribed eating times even if they have eaten a short while before; normal weight individuals tend to eat only when they feel hungry and this is relatively independent of clock time. However, we cannot simply infer that this increased sensitivity to external cues is what causes some people to become obese—it could just as well be an effect of obesity. So what other likely causes are there? Differences in basal metabolic rate (how fast we burn up our body's energy stores) largely determine our body weight and these differences seem to be hereditary (Carlson, 1992).

The role of psychological variables, such as lack of impulse control, poor ability to delay gratification and maladaptive eating styles (primarily eating too fast), are often suggested as causes of obesity. Also, unhappiness and depression seem to be the effects of obesity, rather than the cause.

Classification of eating disorders

The role of complex psychological variables has been studied much more extensively in relation to anorexia nervosa and bulimia nervosa. Both of these, but not obesity, are included in the category of 'eating disorders' in DSM-IV (1994)—the formal classification of mental and behavioural disorders published by the American Psychiatric Association. In the World Health Organization's classification system (9ICD-10, 1992), anorexia and bulimia are categorised under 'behavioural syndromes associated with physiological disturbances and physical factors'. While obesity is included in an appendix called 'Other conditions from ICD-10 often associated with mental and behavioural disorders', anorexia nervosa (literally, 'nervous lack of appetite') is characterised by deliberate weight loss, induced and sustained by the patient. It occurs most commonly in adolescent girls and young women, but adolescent boys and young men may also be affected, as may children approaching puberty and older women up to the menopause. It is associated with a self-perception of being too fat, an intrusive dread of fatness and flabbiness of the body shape (Figure 5.4 ?? where is this??), and the patient imposes a low weight threshold on themselves. There is a serious risk of people who do not receive treatment becoming chronically ill or even dying.

Childhood obesity

One in ten six-year-olds is obese and the total number of obese children has doubled since 1982. So is this just harmless puppy fat or something more serious? Children have high energy requirements because they are growing. A well-balanced and nutritious diet is essential for their development. However, like adults, if they take in more energy in the form of food than they use up, the extra energy is stored in their bodies as fat. It is estimated that up to 15 per cent of children in the UK are overweight or obese. If a child becomes obese their body processes can change; some of these processes may be difficult or impossible to alter in adulthood.

A serious problem

Many cases of childhood obesity is a problem of parenting; parents who bribe or reward children with sweets, or who ply children with sweet stuff in the hope of receiving love in return, are sowing the seeds of obesity. Children who are overweight tend to grow up into adults who are overweight. They therefore have a higher risk of developing serious health problems in later life, including heart attack and stroke, type 2 diabetes, bowel cancer, and high blood pressure. The risk of health problems increases the more overweight a person becomes. Being overweight as a child can also cause psychological distress. Teasing about their appearance affects children's confidence and self-esteem and can lead to isolation and depression. The number of overweight and obese children in the UK has risen steadily over the past twenty years and is now a major health concern.

Why are more children overweight?

Very few children become overweight because of an underlying medical problem. Children are more likely to be obese if their parents are obese but genetic factors are thought to be less significant than the fact that families tend to share eating and activity habits. In other words, most children put on excess weight because their lifestyles include an unhealthy diet and a lack of physical activity. It is certainly easier than ever before for children to become overweight. High calorie foods, such as fast food and confectionery, are abundant, relatively cheap and heavily promoted specifically at children. Exercise is no longer a regular part of everyone's day—some children never walk or cycle to school, or play any kind of sport. And it is not unusual for children to spend hours in front of a television or computer. The National Diet and Nutrition Survey (2000) found that 40–69 per cent of children over the age of six spend less than the recommended minimum of one hour a day doing moderate intensity physical activity.

What is a healthy weight for a child?

Parents often protest that their child has temporary 'puppy fat' and is not genuinely overweight. In adults, a simple formula (the body mass index, or BMI) is used to work out whether a person is the right weight for their height. But BMI alone is not an appropriate measure for children—it has to be used alongside charts that take into account the child's rate of growth, sex and age—and is best interpreted with the help of the GP, practice nurse or, if the condition is giving serious concern, the dietician. It is possible to measure the proportion of body weight that is made up of fat. Generally speaking, a child's weight is classed as obese when their body weight is more than 25 per cent fat in boys and 32 per cent in girls.

Obesity and bullying

Although in adults it not infrequently found that 'secondary benefits' (Chapter 2, p. ?) may create obstacles in enabling people to achieve their desired outcomes, this is seldom the case with overweight or obese children. Children who are seen to be fat by their peers are inevitably subjected to bullying in the form of verbal and often physical abuse. There are seldom any secondary benefits to be gained from this situation. Diets are difficult to maintain and almost impossible to monitor in school children. What is possible, in a large percentage of such cases, is to bring about basic changes in eating habits. The five rules of good eating given while the subject is in hypnosis have proved to be very successful and long lasting:

Rule One: You will eat only when you are genuinely hungry. You know the meaning of genuinely hungry. You will eat only when you are genuinely hungry.

Rule Two: When your hunger is satisfied you will stop eating. When your hunger is satisfied you will stop eating. Even when there may still be food on your plate. Even when there may be food before you. When your hunger is satisfied you will stop eating.

Rule Three: You will eat only those foods that you know are good for you. You will not eat those foods which you know are not good for you. That includes all those foods which we have discussed today. You will eat only those foods that you know are good for you.

Rule Four: You will restrict your calorie intake to 1500 calories per day. You will restrict your calorie intake to 1500 calories per day.

Rule Five: Following these rules of good eating, you will lose a minimum of three to four pounds of ugly unwanted fat every week.

No matter where you go, no matter what company you are in, you will keep these rules of good eating until such times as you achieve your desired weight. Having achieved your desired weight, you will continue to follow these rules of good eating.

Because it is your will and desire to take control of your eating habits and lose weight you will be happy to follow these rules of good eating and feel good about it.

The chocoholic

Sarah was a typical English rose; peaches and cream complexion; a lovely full figure but by no means fat; age about eighteen years; tall for a girl—about five foot seven or eight. As I entered her name and address in my case book, I wondered what could be her problem. She looked as near to a perfect specimen as I had seen. No sign of stress in her lovely face. She looked happy and relaxed. 'What can I do for you?' I asked. 'I'm a chocoholic.' I was amazed. Her complexion was perfect as was her figure. 'How much chocolate do you eat?' 'I eat it all the time.' 'Isn't that a bit of a generalisation? What else do you eat?' 'Not a lot.' 'I mean, your ordinary meals, lunch, dinner, that sort of thing.' 'Yes.' 'You mean that you eat chocolate at those times as well.' 'Yes.' 'What about at work?' 'Yes.' 'What sort of job do you do?' 'I work in my dad's shop.' 'What sort of shop?' 'Well, he has two shops, a confectionery and pastry shop and next door he has a sweet shop. I work in both of them.' 'So you have an unlimited supply of chocolate?' 'Right.' 'And you take advantage of that?' 'All the time.' To say that I was surprised was a gross understatement. Not because of what she was doing but of what I was seeing before me. In theory she should have been fat and spotty. Her complexion was perfect. Her figure was excellent. She was 'chocolate box ' beautiful. Having tested her imagination and visualisation with the 'lemon test', I used the Elman technique induction and direct suggestion to remove the need, desire and craving for chocolate and the post-hypnotic suggestion: 'From the time I tell you to wake up again today you will not ever eat chocolate again.' She had three sessions but never ate chocolate after the first session.

Never make assumptions

About three months later this girl walked into my office. I was surprised to see her again. 'Hello Sarah; what can I do for you this time?' I asked. She smiled, 'I'm not Sarah, that's my sister. I'm Jane and I'm a chocoholic.' It was amazing. The likeness was perfect. I could not have known one from the other even if they had been side by side. 'How is your sister?' 'Oh she's fine. She's not had any chocolate since.' I have heard many experts in the field say that there is always something different between even the closest twins but these two must be the closest possible to identical. I had also heard it said that the first born, if only by a few minutes, was always dominant. I was able to see for myself that these two statements were probably true. As Jane sat in her chair, I asked her to put her hands on her lap and as she did so, I saw that her fingernails were bitten far down. I knew that this was not the case with Sarah. I asked Jane, 'Was Sarah the first born?' 'Yes, but only by five minutes.' 'And is she the bossy one?' 'You can bet on it.' 'And I think that that winds you up a lot?' 'All the time.'

8

Disorders of personality

Major depressive disorder

Because a person is complaining of being depressed, it does not mean that they are suffering major depressive disorder. In most cases clients complaining of depression are really suffering from reactive depression. In other words they have recently suffered an emotional trauma: a bereavement, loss of a job, divorce, serious financial loss, business failure or some such emotional disaster. In these cases hypnotherapy can be very effective in helping sufferers back to emotional health. At least one of the following three abnormal moods which significantly interfere with the person's life must be present if they are suffering major depressive disorder. The following diagnostics are quoted with the permission of the World Health Organization.

Mood symptoms of major depressive disorder:

Extreme depressed mood:

Sadness is usually a normal reaction to loss. However, in major depressive disorder, sadness is abnormal because it:

- Persists continuously for at least two weeks
- Causes marked functional impairment
- Causes disabling psychological symptoms (e.g. apathy, morbid preoccupation with worthlessness, suicidal ideation, or psychotic symptoms).

The sadness in this disorder is often described as a depressed, hopeless and discouraged. This sadness may be denied at first.

Many victims complain of bodily aches and pains, rather than admitting to their true feelings of sadness.

The loss of interest and pleasure in this disorder is a reduced capacity to experience pleasure which in its most extreme form is called anhedonia and the resulting lack of motivation can be quite crippling.

Major depressive disorder causes the following physical symptoms:

Abnormal appetite:

- Most depressed patients experience loss of appetite and weight loss. The opposite, excessive eating and weight gain, occurs in a minority of depressed patients. Changes in weight can be significant.

Abnormal sleep:

- Most depressed patients experience difficulty falling asleep, frequent awakenings during the night or very early morning awakening. The opposite, excessive sleeping, occurs in a minority of depressed patients.

Fatigue or loss of energy:

- Profound fatigue and lack of energy usually are very prominent and disabling.

Agitation or slowing:

- Psychomotor retardation (an actual physical slowing of speech, movement and thinking) or psychomotor agitation (observable pacing and physical restlessness) often are present in severe major depressive disorder.

Major depressive disorder causes the following cognitive symptoms:

Abnormal self-reproach or inappropriate guilt:

- This disorder usually causes a marked lowering of self-esteem and self-confidence with increased thoughts of pessimism, hopelessness and helplessness. In the extreme, the person may feel excessively and unreasonably guilty.

    The 'negative thinking' caused by depression can become extremely dangerous as it can eventually lead to extremely self-defeating or suicidal behaviour.

Abnormal poor concentration or indecisiveness:

- Poor concentration is often an early symptom of this disorder. The depressed person quickly becomes mentally fatigued when asked to read, study or solve complicated problems.

    Marked forgetfulness often accompanies this disorder. As it worsens, this memory loss can be easily mistaken for early senility (dementia).

Abnormal morbid thoughts of death (not just fear of dying) or suicide:

- The symptom most highly correlated with suicidal behaviour in depression is hopelessness.

Associated features—anxiety:

- 80 to 90 per cent of individuals with major depressive disorder also have anxiety symptoms (e.g. anxiety, obsessive preoccupations, panic attacks, phobias, and excessive health concerns). Separation anxiety may be prominent in children.

    About one third of individuals with major depressive disorder also have a full-blown anxiety disorder (usually either panic disorder, obsessive-compulsive disorder, or social phobia).

    Anxiety in a person with major depression leads to a

poorer response to treatment, poorer social and work function, greater likelihood of becoming chronic and an increased risk of suicidal behaviour.

Eating disorders:

- Individuals with anorexia nervosa and bulimia nervosa often develop major depressive disorder.

Psychosis:

- Mood congruent delusions or hallucinations may accompany severe major depressive disorder.

Substance abuse:

- The combination of major depressive disorder and substance abuse is common (especially alcohol and cocaine).
  Alcohol or street drugs are often mistakenly used as a remedy for depression. However, this abuse of alcohol or street drugs actually worsens major depressive disorder.
  Depression may also be a consequence of drug or alcohol withdrawal and is commonly seen after cocaine and amphetamine use.

Medical illness:

- 25 per cent of individuals with severe, chronic medical illness (e.g. diabetes, myocardial infarction, carcinomas and stroke) develop depression.
  About 5 per cent of individuals initially diagnosed as having major depressive disorder are subsequently found to have another medical illness which was the cause of their depression.
  Medical conditions often causing depression are:
  - *Endocrine disorders*: hypothyroidism, hyperparathyroidism, Cushing's disease, and diabetes mellitus.
  - *Neurological disorders*: multiple sclerosis, Parkinson's disease, migraine, various forms of epilepsy, encephalitis, brain tumours.

- *Medications*: many medications can cause depression, especially antihypertensive agents such as calcium channel blockers, beta blockers, analgesics and some anti-migraine medications.

Mortality

Up to 15 per cent of patients with severe major depressive disorder die by suicide. Over age 55, there is a four-fold increase in death rate; 10–25 per cent of patients with major depressive disorder have pre-existing dysthymic disorder. These 'double depressions' (i.e. dysthymia + major depressive disorder) have a poorer prognosis.

Gender

Males and females are equally affected by major depressive disorder prior to puberty. After puberty, this disorder is twice as common in females as in males. The highest rates for this disorder are in the 25- to 44-year-old age group.

Onset and course

Psychological stress:

- Stress appears to play a prominent role in triggering the first one or two episodes of this disorder, but not in subsequent episodes.
- *Duration*:
  - An average episode lasts about nine months
- *Course*:
  - Course is variable. Some people have isolated episodes that are separated by many years, whereas others have clusters of episodes, and still others have increasingly frequent episodes as they grow older.
    About 20 per cent of individuals with this disorder have a chronic course.

Recurrence

The risk of recurrence is about 70 per cent at five year follow-up and at least 80 per cent at eight year follow-up.

After the first episode of major depressive disorder, there is a 50–60 per cent chance of having a second episode, and a 5–10 per cent chance of having a manic episode (i.e. developing bipolar I disorder). After the second episode, there is a 70 per cent chance of having a third. After the third episode, there a 90 per cent chance of having a fourth.

The greater number of previous episodes is an important risk factor for recurrence.

Recovery

For patients with severe major depressive disorder, 76 per cent on antidepressant therapy recover, whereas only 18 per cent on placebo recover. For these severely depressed patients, significantly more recover on antidepressant therapy than on interpersonal psychotherapy. For these same patients, cognitive therapy has been shown to be no more effective than placebo.

Poor outcome

Poor outcome in major depressive disorder is associated with the following:

- Inadequate treatment
- Severe initial symptoms
- Early age of onset
- Greater number of previous episodes
- Only partial recovery after one year
- Having another severe mental disorder (e.g. alcohol dependency, cocaine dependency)
- Severe chronic medical illness
- Family dysfunction .

Familial pattern and genetics

There is strong evidence that major depression is, in part, a genetic disorder:

- Individuals who have parents or siblings with major depressive disorder have a 1.5–3 times higher risk of developing this disorder.

- The concordance for major depression in monozygotic twins is substantially higher than it is in dizygotic twins. However, the concordance in monozygotic twins is in the order of about 50 per cent, suggesting that factors other than genetic factors are also involved.

- Children adopted away at birth from biological parents who have a depressive illness carry the same high risk as a child not adopted away, even if they are raised in a family where no depressive illness exists.

Interestingly, families having major depressive disorder have an increased risk of developing alcoholism and attention deficit hyperactivity disorder.

Acute and transient psychotic disorder

Systematic clinical information that would provide definitive guidance on the classification of acute psychotic disorders is not yet available, and the limited data and clinical tradition that must therefore be used instead do not give rise to concepts that can be clearly defined and separated from each other. In the absence of a tried and tested multiaxial system, the method used to avoid diagnostic confusion is to construct a diagnostic sequence that reflects the order of priority given to selected key features of the disorder. The order of priority used here is:

(a) an acute onset (within two weeks) as the defining feature of the whole group;

(b)   the presence of typical syndromes; and

(c)   the presence of associated acute stress.

The classification is nevertheless arranged so that those who do not agree with this order of priority can still identify acute psychotic disorders with each of these specified features.

It is also recommended that whenever possible a further subdivision of onset be used, if applicable, for all the disorders of this group. Acute onset is defined as a change from a state without psychotic features to a clearly abnormal psychotic state, within a period of two weeks or less. There is some evidence that acute onset is associated with a good outcome, and it may be that the more abrupt the onset, the better the outcome. It is therefore recommended that, whenever appropriate, abrupt onset (within 48 hours or less) be specified.

The typical syndromes that have been selected are first, the rapidly changing and variable state, called here 'polymorphic', that has been given prominence in acute psychotic states in several countries, and second, the presence of typical schizophrenic symptoms.

Associated acute stress can also be specified, with a fifth character if desired, in view of its traditional linkage with acute psychosis. The limited evidence available, however, indicates that a substantial proportion of acute psychotic disorders arise without associated stress, and provision has therefore been made for the presence or the absence of stress to be recorded. Associated acute stress is taken to mean that the first psychotic symptoms occur within about two weeks of one or more events that would be regarded as stressful to most people in similar circumstances, within the culture of the person concerned. Typical events would be bereavement, unexpected loss of partner or job, marriage, or the psychological trauma of combat, terrorism and torture. Long-standing difficulties or problems should not be included as a source of stress in this context.

Complete recovery usually occurs within two to three months, often within a few weeks or even days, and only a small proportion of patients with these disorders develop persistent and disabling states. Unfortunately, the present state of knowledge does not allow the early prediction of that small proportion of patients who will not recover rapidly.

Dependent personality disorder

Basic principles

Patients with dependent personality disorder may make a dramatic appeal for caretaking, with urgent and inappropriate demands for immediate attention to their medical complaints, which have an exaggerated quality. If they fail to receive a prompt response, they may erupt in angry outbursts that threaten important emotional ties, including that with the physician. Since illness provides secondary gains in the form of caretaking and attention, such patients tend to be passive participants in the healing partnership rather than seeking active solutions.

The well-known oral characteristics of dependent persons may be expressed in food, alcohol, and drug problems. The physician must be especially alert to the possibility of abuse of sedatives, hypnotics, tranquilisers, and analgesics. Patients with dependent personality disorder are overly compliant in their acceptance of medical treatment and may search for gratification of their unmet dependency needs by seeking unnecessary procedures while minimising the associated hazards.

To patients with dependent personality disorder, physical illness represents the wish for the continuous soothing ministrations of the physician and also embodies a fear of abandonment. Being physically ill, with its considerable discomforts, may be equated with a lack of love or interest, and patients blame 'bad' caretakers for their distress. The physician should provide reassurance and convey an impression of being available and accessible to the patient but should be careful to explain clearly and firmly the realistic limits of such availability. The physician can provide help in other ways, e.g. co-ordinating support services and instituting flexible appointment scheduling, in which the patient assumes some responsibility for establishing the timing of appointments.

Physicians treating these patients must guard against 'burnout' and the hostile rejection that may be aroused by these patients' strong dependency needs. The patient's exaggerated compliance with the treatment regimen may lead to over-utilisation of medical care systems and is another item that healthcare professionals need to be aware of. Other members of the healthcare team, including nurses and physical therapists, may play an important role in communicating the physician's interest and concern and in alleviating physical discomfort, so that the burden of meeting dependency needs is distributed throughout the team rather than being focused exclusively on any one member.

In general, psychoactive drugs must only be prescribed for clear indications. The complications and the frequency of polydrug abuse, especially sedative-hypnotic drugs, in patients with personality disorders are enormous. So are overdoses. Although a small number of patients who have personality disorders and secondary depression or panic disorders may be helped by antidepressants, many thousands of personality disordered patients make serious suicide attempts with antidepressants every year. On many occasions those with personality disorders need someone to remind them that anxiety and insomnia are non-fatal, self-limiting maladies; they need clinicians who can bear their painful emotions and who do not simply anaesthetise them. So often when one tries to treat a personality disordered patient with medication, the no-win relationship asserts itself, and medication becomes a bone of contention between patient and therapist.

In personality disorders, the placebo effect of medication for both good and ill is immense. New drugs, whatever their pharmacological composition, are more widely used and more magically useful in personality disorders than are old drugs. Time-controlled studies show that if new drugs fail their early promise and lead to abuse and overdose, then, their magic wears off, and they become old drugs. The use of safe, honestly used, non-psychoactive pharmacological agents, such as L-tryptophan or vitamins, for their symbolic value, for their evidence that the doctor cares, and for giving the patient a talisman is, however, sometimes helpful in managing patients with personality disorders.

Hospitalisation

Situations of severe loss or intense effect in these patients should lead the therapist to consider protective measures such as hospitalisation, in which the patient can be contained to some extent and definitive therapy for Axis I symptoms carried out in a controlled setting.

Psychosocial treatment

Basic principles

As with many of the other personality disorders, patients with this diagnosis are unlikely to seek treatment. They may, however, wish to explore reasons for lack of social or vocational success, and may suffer considerable loss when an important figure leaves them in one way or another.

Referrals of dependent patients within a consultation-liaison framework are common; however, many of these patients' characteristics are related to their medical illness or the hospital setting, and do not fill DSM-III criteria.

One pitfall in the treatment of dependent personalities occurs when the therapist challenges a pathological but dependent relationship, for example when the therapist insists that a wife-beater's wife seek help from the police. The patient may become increasingly anxious and unable to co-operate in therapy and feel torn between the therapist and the risk of losing a pathological external relationship. In short, great respect must be shown for a dependent patient's feelings of attachment, no matter how pathological those feelings seem to the observer.

Individual psychotherapy

Long-term psychotherapy is the treatment of choice and should focus on the patient's exaggerated fears of damaging others or oneself by pursuing autonomy and becoming one's own person.

An important early therapeutic task is acceptance by the therapist of much of the same dependence that the patient feels toward others in his or her life. The symptoms and psychodynamics can then be discussed at first hand, rather than in the patient's reports of feelings about others. The therapist's support of the patient's individuation from others (and now from the therapist as well) should include practical issues such as jobs and housing. Anxiety and depression may result, and should be taken seriously since severely dependent patients may harbour a potential for overwhelming despondency or rage against the self or others.

Termination is a delicate task, and should be a joint decision. The therapist should be flexible, allowing the patient to return as needed.

Group therapy

Patients with this condition tend to improve with supportive, insight-oriented individual or group therapy.

Behaviour therapy

The treatment of dependent personality traits can be very successful. Sometimes behaviour therapies, especially assertiveness training, are the quickest road to interpersonal adjustment for the dependent person.

The nomenclature of these acute disorders is as uncertain as their nosological status, but an attempt has been made to use simple and familiar terms. Psychotic disorder is used as a term of convenience for all the members of this group with an additional qualifying term indicating the major defining feature of each separate type as it appears in the sequence noted above.

Diagnostic guidelines

None of the disorders in the group satisfies the criteria for either manic or depressive episodes, although emotional changes and individual affective symptoms may be prominent from time to time.

These disorders are also defined by the absence of organic causation, such as states of concussion, delirium, or dementia. Perplexity, preoccupation, and inattention to the immediate conversation are often present, but if they are so marked or persistent as to suggest delirium or dementia of organic cause, the diagnosis should be delayed until investigation or observation has clarified this point. Similarly, disorders in F23 should not be diagnosed in the presence of obvious intoxication by drugs or alcohol. However, a recent minor increase in the consumption of, for instance, alcohol or marijuana, with no evidence of severe intoxication or disorientation, should not rule out the diagnosis of one of these acute psychotic disorders.

It is important to note that the 48-hour and the two-week criteria are not put forward as the times of maximum severity and disturbance, but as times by which the psychotic symptoms have become obvious and disruptive of at least some aspects of daily life and work. The peak disturbance may be reached later in both instances; the symptoms and disturbance have only to be obvious by the stated times, in the sense that they will usually have brought the patient into contact with some form of helping or medical agency. Prodromal periods of anxiety, depression, social withdrawal or mildly abnormal behaviour do not qualify for inclusion in these periods of time.

Five (or more) of the following symptoms have been present during the same two-week period and represent a change from previous functioning; at least one of the symptoms is either (1) depressed mood or (2) loss of interest or pleasure.

Note: Do not include symptoms that are clearly due to a general medical condition, mood-incongruent delusions or hallucinations, depressed mood most of the day, nearly every day, as indicated by either subjective report (e.g. feels sad or empty) or observation made by others (e.g. appears tearful).

Note: In children and adolescents, can be irritable mood.

- Markedly diminished interest or pleasure in all, or almost all, activities most of the day, nearly every day (as indicated by either subjective account or observation made by others)

- Significant weight loss when not dieting or weight gain (e.g. a change of more than 5 per cent of body weight in a month), or decrease or increase in appetite nearly every day **Note**: In children, consider failure to make expected weight gains. Insomnia or hypersomnia nearly every day

- Psychomotor agitation or retardation nearly every day (observable by others, not merely subjective feelings of restlessness or being slowed down)

- Fatigue or loss of energy nearly every day

- Feelings of worthlessness or excessive or inappropriate guilt (which may be delusional) nearly every day (not merely self-reproach or guilt about being sick)

- Diminished ability to think or concentrate, or indecisiveness, nearly every day (either by subjective account or as observed by others)

- Recurrent thoughts of death (not just fear of dying), recurrent suicidal ideation without a specific plan, or a suicide attempt or a specific plan for committing suicide

- The symptoms do not meet criteria for a mixed episode

- The symptoms cause clinically significant distress or impairment in social, occupational, or other important areas of functioning

- The symptoms are not due to the direct physiological effects of a substance (e.g. a drug of abuse, a medication) or a general medical condition (e.g. hypothyroidism)

- The symptoms are not better accounted for by bereavement, i.e. after the loss of a loved one, the symptoms persist for longer than two months or are characterised by marked functional impairment, morbid preoccupation with worthlessness, suicidal ideation, psychotic symptoms, or psychomotor retardation.

Manic episode

- A distinct period of abnormally and persistently elevated, expansive, or irritable mood, lasting at least one week (or any duration if hospitalisation is necessary)
- During the period of mood disturbance, three (or more) of the following symptoms have persisted (four if the mood is only irritable) and have been present to a significant degree:
  - Inflated self-esteem or grandiosity
  - Decreased need for sleep (e.g. feels rested after only three hours of sleep)
  - More talkative than usual or pressure to keep talking
  - Flight of ideas or subjective experience that thoughts are racing
  - Distractibility (i.e. attention too easily drawn to unimportant or irrelevant external stimuli)
  - Increase in goal-directed activity (either socially, at work or school, or sexually) or psychomotor agitation
  - Excessive involvement in pleasurable activities that have a high potential for painful consequences (e.g. engaging in unrestrained buying sprees, sexual indiscretions, or foolish business investments)
  - The symptoms do not meet criteria for a mixed episode
  - The mood disturbance is sufficiently severe to cause marked impairment in occupational functioning or in usual social activities or relationships with others, or to necessitate hospitalisation to prevent harm to self or others, or there are psychotic features
  - The symptoms are not due to the direct physiological effects of a substance (e.g. a drug of abuse, a medication, or other treatment) or a general medical condition (e.g. hyperthyroidism).

Mixed episode

- The criteria are met both for a manic episode and for a major depressive episode (except for duration) nearly every day during at least a one-week period
- The mood disturbance is sufficiently severe to cause marked impairment in occupational functioning or in usual social activities or relationships with others, or to necessitate hospitalisation to prevent harm to self or others, or there are psychotic features
- The symptoms are not due to the direct physiological effects of a substance (e.g. a drug of abuse, a medication, or other treatment) or a general medical condition (e.g. hyper-thyroidism).

Hypomanic episode

- A distinct period of persistently elevated, expansive, or irritable mood, lasting throughout at least four days, that is clearly different from the usual nondepressed mood.
- During the period of mood disturbance, three (or more) of the following symptoms have persisted (four if the mood is only irritable) and have been present to a significant degree:
  - Inflated self-esteem or grandiosity
  - Decreased need for sleep (e.g. feels rested after only three hours of sleep)
  - More talkative than usual or pressure to keep talking
  - Flight of ideas or subjective experience that thoughts are racing
  - Distractibility (i.e. attention too easily drawn to unimportant or irrelevant external stimuli)
  - Increase in goal-directed activity (either socially, at work or school, or sexually) or psychomotor agitation
  - Excessive involvement in pleasurable activities that have a high potential for painful consequences (e.g. the

person engages in unrestrained buying sprees, sexual indiscretions, or foolish business investments)

- The episode is associated with an unequivocal change in functioning that is uncharacteristic of the person when not symptomatic
- The disturbance in mood and the change in functioning are observable by others
- The episode is not severe enough to cause marked impairment in social or occupational functioning, or to necessitate hospitalisation, and there are no psychotic features
- The symptoms are not due to the direct physiological effects of a substance (e.g. a drug of abuse, a medication, or other treatment) or a general medical condition (e.g. hyperthyroidism).
  Note: Hypomanic-like episodes that are clearly caused by somatic antidepressant treatment (e.g. medication, electroconvulsive therapy, light therapy) should not count toward a diagnosis of bipolar II disorder.

Obsessive compulsive disorder (OCD)

The most common features of OCD are obsessional thoughts and compulsive behaviour. Obsessional thoughts are distressing, repetitive thoughts which you know are your own (unlike hallucinations) but cannot ignore; some people describe these as being like a 'stuck record'. Compulsions are ritual actions or mental processes which you feel compelled to repeat in order to relieve anxiety and temporarily stop obsessional thoughts. For example, you may have an obsessional thought that your hands are dirty and repeatedly wash them over and over again. Obsessive thoughts and compulsive rituals can take up many hours of each day. In its most severe form, OCD can prevent you from completing even simple daily tasks, such as washing the dishes.

What are the symptoms of OCD?

Not all obsessive thoughts and compulsive behaviours are symptoms of a mental health problem. Most of us have worries, doubts and superstitious beliefs. It is only when thoughts and behaviour make no sense, cause distress or become excessive that help should be sought.

OCD symptoms can occur at any stage of life. A sufferer from OCD may also feel anxious and depressed, and believe he/she is the only person with such irrational and obsessive thoughts. Unfortunately, such feelings can create a fear of telling anyone or asking for help, which only delays diagnosis and treatment. Having OCD should not be seen as a sign of weakness or as lacking willpower because of an inability to stop these thoughts and behaviours. Symptoms of OCD are also seen in other brain disorders such as Tourette's syndrome.

Most common obsessions and compulsions

Obsessions	Compulsions
Fear of contamination	Cleaning and washing
Fear of causing harm to someone else	Checking
Fear of making a mistake	Arranging and organising
Fear of behaving unacceptably	Collecting and hoarding
Need for symmetry or exactness	Counting and repeating
Excessive doubt	

What causes OCD?

There are different theories about why OCD develops. It can be based on previous experiences, especially during childhood. The type of personality may also be important—perfectionists seem to be more prone to this problem. OCD has been linked to increased activity in certain parts of the brain and some experts think low levels of a brain chemical called serotonin may be involved, although others disagree. Stress does not cause OCD, but a stressful event such as birth, death or divorce may act as a trigger.

9

Extract from *A Dream of Genes*

This final chapter is published with permission of Dr Bruce Lipton, PhD.

Dr Lipton was born in Mount Kisco, New York in 1944. He gained his PhD in developmental cell biology in 1971 and has held teaching positions and professorships in anatomy and biology. He member of the board of the American Institute of Hypnotherapy. This chapter is an extract from his video *A Dream of Genes*.

A new view of biology

Francis Bacon defined the mission of modern science shortly after the onset of the scientific revolution (1543). Accordingly, the purpose of science was 'to dominate and control Nature'. To accomplish that goal, scientists had to first acquire knowledge of what 'controls' an organism's structure and function (behaviour). Concepts founded in the principles of Newtonian physics defined the experimental approach to this quest. These principles stipulate that the Universe is a 'Physical mechanism' comprised of parts (matter); there is no attention given to the invisible 'energy'. In this (Newtonian) world view, the only thing of importance is 'matter'. Consequently, modern science is preoccupied with materialism.

The materialist's way

The way to understand how a finely tuned mechanism works is to disassemble it and analysis all of the component 'parts' and how they interact; defective part(s) in a malfunctioning organism can be identified and either repaired or replaced with 'manufactured' parts (drugs, engineered genes, prosthetic devices, etc). Knowledge of the body's mechanism would enable scientists to determine how the organism works and how to 'control the organism by altering its "parts"'.

Biologists were preoccupied with taking organisms apart and studying their cells for the first half of this century. Subsequently, cells were disassembled and their molecular 'parts' catalogued and characterised. Cells are comprised of four types of large (macro-) molecules: proteins; polysaccharides (sugars); nucleic acids (gene stuff); lipids (fats).

The component parts

The name 'protein' means 'primary element' (proteios, Gr.) for proteins are the primary components of all plant and animal cells. A human is made of a million different proteins. Proteins are linear 'chains', whose molecular 'links' are comprised of amino acid molecules. Each of the twenty different amino acids has a unique shape, so that when linked together in a chain, the resulting proteins fold into elaborate three-dimensional 'wire sculptures'. The protein sculpture's pattern is determined by the sequence of its amino acid links. The balancing of electromagnetic charges along the protein's chain serves to control the 'final' shape of the sculpture. The unique shape of a protein sculpture is referred to as its 'confirmation'. In the manner of a lock and key, protein sculptures complement the shape of environmental molecules (that include other proteins). When proteins interlock with the complementary environmental molecules, they assemble into complex structures (similar to the way cogged 'gears' intermesh to make a watch).

Protein pathways

When proteins chemically couple with other molecules, they change the distribution of electromagnetic charges in the protein. Changes in 'charge' cause the protein to change its shape. Therefore, upon coupling with chemicals, a protein will shift its shape from one conformation to another. A protein generates 'motion' as it changes shape. A protein's movement can be harnessed to do 'work'. Groups of interacting proteins that work together in carrying out a specific function are referred to as 'pathways'. The activities of specific protein pathways provide for digestion, excretion, respiration, reproduction, and all of the other physiologic 'functions' employed by living organisms.

Proteins provide for the organism's structure and function, but random protein actions cannot provide for 'life'. Scientists needed to identify the mechanism that 'integrates' protein functions to allow for the complex behaviours. Their search was linked to the fact that proteins are labile (opposite of stabile). Like parts in a car, proteins 'wear out' when they are used. If an individual protein in a pathway wears out and is not replaced then the action of the pathway will stop. To resume function, the protein must be replaced. Consequently, behavioural functions were thought to be controlled by 'regulating' the presence or absence of proteins comprising the pathways. The source of replacement protein parts is related to 'memory' factors that provide for heredity...the passing on of 'character'.

Hereditary factors

The search for the hereditary factors that controlled protein synthesis led to DNA, served as a molecular 'blueprint', that defined amino acid sequences comprising a protein. The DNA blueprint for each protein is referred to as a gene. Since proteins define the character of an organism and the proteins' structures are encoded in the DNA, biologists established the dogma known as the 'Primacy of DNA'. In this context, primacy means 'first level of control'. It was concluded that DNA 'controls' the structure and behaviour of living organisms. Since DNA 'determines' the character of an organism, then it is appropriate to acknowledge the concept of 'Genetic Determination', the idea that the structure and behaviour of an organism are defined by its genes.

Science's materialist-reductionist-determinist philosophy led to the Human Genome Project, the multibillion-dollar program to map all of the genes. Once this is accomplished, it is assumed that we can use that knowledge to repair or replace 'defective' genes and in the process, realise science's mission of 'controlling' the expression of an organism.

Dispelling the myth of genes

Since 1953, biologists have assumed that DNA 'controls' life. In multicellular animals, the organ that 'controls' life is known as the brain. Since genes are presumed to control cellular life, and genes are contained in the cell's nucleus, the nucleus would be expected to be the equivalent of the cell's 'brain'. It has now been discovered that this is not the case.

If the brain is removed from any organism, the immediate and necessary consequence of that action is death of the organism. Removing the cell's nucleus, referred to as enucleation, would be tantamount to removing the cell's brain. Although enucleation should result in the immediate death of the cell, enucleated cells may continue to survive and exhibit a 'regulated' control of their biological processes. In fact cells can live for two or more months without a nucleus. Clearly, the assumption that genes 'control' cell behaviour is wrong.

As is described by Nijhout, (X) genes are 'not self-emergent', that is genes cannot turn themselves on or off. If genes cannot control their own expression, how can they control the behaviour of the cell? Nijhout further emphasises that genes are regulated by 'environmental signals'. *Consequently, it is the environment that controls gene expression.* Rather than endorsing the Primacy of DNA, we must acknowledge the 'Primacy of the Environment'.

Cell survival

Cells 'read' their environment, assess the information and then select appropriate behaviour programs to maintain their survival. The fact that data is integrated, processed and used to make a calculated behavioural response emphasises the existence of a 'brain' equivalent in the cell. Where is the cell's brain? The answer is to be found in bacteria, the most primitive organisms on Earth. The many processes and functions of this unicellular life form are highly integrated; consequently, it must have a brain equivalent. Cytologically, these organisms do not contain any organelles (diminutive of 'organs') such as nuclei, mitochondria, golgi bodies, etc. The only organised structure in these primitive life forms is their 'cell membrane', also known as their plasmalemma. The cell membrane once thought to be like a permeable Saran Wrap that holds the cytoplasm together, actually provides for the bacterium's digestive, respiratory, excretory and integumentary (skin) systems. It also serves as the cell's 'brain'.

Integral membrane proteins

The cell membrane is primarily composed of phospholipids and proteins. Phospholipids, which resemble lollipops with two sticks, are arranged in a crystalline bilayer. The membrane resembles a bread and butter sandwich, wherein the lipid 'sticks' form the central butter layer. The phospholipids bilayer forms a skin-like barrier which separates the external environment from the internal cytoplasm.

Built into the membrane are special proteins called integral membrane proteins (IMPs). IMPs look like olives in the membrane's bread and butter sandwich. There are two classes of IMPs: receptors and effectors. Receptors are the cell's 'sense' organs, the equivalents of eyes, ears, nose, etc. When a receptor recognises and binds to a signal, it responds by changing its conformation. Conventional biology stipulates that receptors only respond to 'matter' (molecules), a belief consistent with the Newtonian view of the Universe as a 'matter machine'.

A Quantum Universe

Leading edge contemporary cell research has transcended conventional Newtonian physics and is now soundly based upon a Universe created out of energy as defined by quantum physics. This new physics emphasises energetics over materialism, substitutes holism for reductionism and recognises uncertainty in place of determinism. Consequently, we now recognise that receptors respond to energy signals as well as to molecular signals.

Conventional medicine has consistently ignored research published in its own mainstream scientific journals, research that clearly reveals the regulatory influence that electromagnetic fields have on cell physiology. Pulsed electromagnetic fields have been shown to regulate virtually every cell function, including DNA synthesis, RNA synthesis, protein synthesis, cell division, cell differentiation, morphogenesis and neuroendocrine regulation. These findings are relevant for they acknowledge that biological behaviour can be controlled by 'invisible' energy forces, which include *thought*.

Effector and receptor proteins

When activated by its complementary signal, the protein receptor changes its conformation so that it is able to complex with a specific effector protein. Effector proteins carry out cell behaviours. Effector proteins may be enzymes, cytoskeleton elements, protons, ions, and other specific molecules across the 'bread and butter' barrier. Generally, effector proteins are inactive in their resting conformation. However, when the receptor binds to the effector protein, it causes the effector to changes its own conformation from an inactive to an active protein form. This is how an environmental signal activates a cell's behaviour. The activity of effector IMPs generally regulates the behaviours of cytoplasmic protein pathways, like those associated with digestion, excretion, and cell movement. If specific functional proteins are not already present in the cell, activated effector IMPs send a signal to the nucleus and elicit required gene programs.

Receptor IMPs 'see' or are 'aware' of their environment and effector IMPs create physical responses that translate environmental signals into an appropriate biological behaviour. The IMP complexes control behaviour and through their effect upon regulatory proteins these IMPs also control gene expression. The IMP complexes provide the cell with 'awareness' of the environment through physical sensation, which by dictionary definition represents *perception*. Each receptor-effector protein complex collectively constitutes a 'unit of perception'. A biochemical definition of the cell membrane reads as follows:

> *'The membrane is a liquid crystal (phospholipids organization), semiconductor. The only things that can cross the membrane barrier are those brought across by transport IMPs with gates (receptor IMPs) and channels (effector IMPs).'*

This definition is exactly the same as that used to define a computer chip. Recent studies have verified that the cell membrane is in fact an organic homologue of a silicon chip.

Cell as organic processor

Taken in this context, the cell is a self-powered microprocessor. Simply stated, the cell is an organic computer. The operation of the cell can be easily understood by noting its homology to the computer: the 'CPU' (information processing mechanism) is the cell membrane, the keyboard (data entry) is the membrane receptors, the disk (memory) is the nucleus, the screen (data output) is the physical state of the cell. Receptor/effector IMP complexes, the units of 'perception', are equivalent to computational bits.

When new, heretofore unrecognised, 'signals' enter the environment, the cell creates new perception units to respond to them. New perception units require 'new' genes for the IMP proteins. The cell's ability to make new IMP receptors and respond to the new signal with an appropriate survival-oriented response (behaviour) is the foundation of evolution. Cells 'learn' by making new receptors and integrating them with specific effector proteins. Cellular memory is represented by the 'new' genes that code for these proteins. This process enables organisms to survive in ever-changing environments.

This learning/evolution mechanism is employed by the immune system. To the immune cell (T-lymphocyte), invasive antigens (e.g. viruses, bacteria, toxins) represent 'new' environmental signals. T-lymphocytes create protein antibodies that complement and bind to the antigens. Antibodies are 'receptors' for they specifically recognise their antigen 'signal'. Protein antibody structure is encoded in genes (DNA). In making new antibodies, cells 'create' new genes.

A cell's awareness of the environment is reflected in its receptor population. In single-celled organism (bacteria, protozoa and algae), the cell's receptors respond to all survival-related environmental signals. These signals include elements of the physical environment (light, gravity, temperature, salts, minerals, etc), food (nutrients, other organisms), and life-threatening agents (toxins, parasites, predators, etc.).

In multicellular organisms, the cells evolved additional receptors required for 'community' identity and integration. Integration receptors respond to information signals (hormones, growth factors) used to co-ordinate functions in cell communities. A special group of receptors confer 'identity' so that members of the cellular community can collectively respond to a 'central' command. Identity receptors are referred to as 'self receptors', or 'histocompatibility receptors'. Self-receptors are used by the immune system to distinguish 'self' from invasive organism. Organs or tissues cannot be exchanged unless they bear the same self-receptors as the recipient.

When a perception unit recognises an environmental signal, it will activate a cell function. Though there are hundreds of behavioural functions expressed by a cell, all behaviours can be classified as either growth or protection responses. Cells move toward growth signals and away from life-threatening stimuli (protection response). Since a cell cannot move forward and backward at the same time, a cell cannot be in growth and protection at the same time. At the cellular level, growth and protection are mutually exclusive behaviours. This is true for human cells as well. If our tissues and organs perceive a need for protection, they will compromise their growth behaviour. Chronic protection leads to a disruption of the tissue and its function.

Adaptive mutation

What happens if a cell experiences a stressful environment but does not have a gene program (behaviour) to deal with the stress? It is now recognised that cells can 'rewrite' existing gene programs in an effort to overcome the stressful condition. These DNA changes are mutations. Until recently, all mutations were thought to be 'random', meaning that the outcome of the mutation could not be directed. It is now recognised that environmental stimuli can induce 'adaptive' mutations that enable a cell to specifically alter its genes. Furthermore, such mutations may be mediated by an organism's perception of its environment. For example, if an organism 'perceives' a stress that is actually not there, the misperception can actually change the genes to accommodate the 'belief'.

In conclusion

The structures of our bodies are defined by our proteins. Proteins represent the physical complement of the environment. Consequently, our bodies are physical complements of our environment. IMP perception units in the cell's membrane convert the environment into awareness. Reception of environment signals changes protein conformations. The 'movement' generated by protein shape change is harnessed by the cell to do 'work'. Life (animation) results from protein movements which are translated as 'behaviour'.

Cells respond to perception by activating either growth or protection behaviour programs. If the necessary behaviour provided proteins are not present in the cytoplasm, the IMP perception units can activate expression of appropriate genes in the cell's nucleus.

'Perceptions' lie between the environment and cell expression. If perceptions are accurate, the resulting behaviour will be life enhancing. If we operate from 'misperceptions', our behaviour will be inappropriate and will jeopardise our vitality by compromising our health.

References

American Psychiatric Association (1994) *Diagnostic and Statistical Manual* (DSM-IV). World Health Organization, New York

American Psychiatric Association (1992) *Mental and Behavioural Disorders*. World Health Organization, 91CD-10, New York

Barber J, *et al* (1996) *Hypnosis and Suggestion in the Treatment of Pain*. W W Norton, London

Beecher HK (1959) *Measurement of Subjective Responses: Quantitative Effects of Drugs*. Oxford University Press, New York

Beecher HK (1955) The powerful placebo. *J Am Med Ass* **159**: 1602–606

Blacker, Clare (1987) *Depressive Disorder in Primary Care*. British Journal of Psychiatry, London

Bower P, *et al* (2001) The clinical effectiveness of self-help treatments. *Br J Clin Pract* **51**(471): 838–45

Braid J (1899) *Neurypnology*. Redway, London

Cangello VW (1962) Leukemia. *Am J Clin Hypnosis* **4**: 215

Colgan SM, *et al* (1988) Relapse prevention in duodenal ulcer. *Lancet* **1**: 1299

Crabtree A (1993) *Mesmer to Freud*. Yale University Publishing, USA

Culbert *et al* (1994) *Application of Clinical Hypnosis with Children*. John Wiley & Sons, New York

Dixon NF (1971) *Subliminal Suggestion*. McGraw Hill, London

Elliotson Dr (1848) Cure of true case of cancer. *Zoist* (1984) **23**: 312

Elman D (1964) *Hypnotherapy*. Westwood Publishing, Glendale CA

Eysenck HJ (1991) *Psychological Factors in the Prevention of Cancer*. Springer Verlag, New York

Fernando (2002) *Mental Health, Race & Culture*, 2nd edn. Palgrave, Hampshire

Finklestein, Howard (1995) Cancer prevention. *Am J Clin Hypnosis* **25**: 177

French P (1983) *Social Skills for Nurses*. Croom Helm, Kent

Gamble C, Brennan G (2000) *Working with Serious Mental Illness*. Bailliere Tindall, London

Hart C (1999) Modern drug discovery. *Am Sci Soc* **2**: 20–21

Hartland J (1971) *Medical and Dental Hypnosis*. Bailliere Tindall, London

Healey M, Murton J (1986) *Create your Future*. Belmont Press, Ramsgate

Hillgard E (1977) *Divided Consciousness*. John Wiley & Sons, New York

Kai Tiaki (2002) Hypnosis skills enrich nursing practice. *New Zealand Nurse* **8**(6): 9

Kirsch, Sapirstein (1998) *Listening to Prozac but Hearing Placebo. Prevention and Treat ment*, Vol 1. University of Connecticut, New York

Klein, Spiegel (1989) Modulation of gastric acid secretion. *J Gastroenterol* **96**(6): 1383–87

Klerman GL (1987) In: Levine, Lilienfield, eds. *Epidemiology and Health Policy*. Tavistock, New York

Kohen D, Kuttner L (1986) *Applications of Clinical Hypnosis with Children*. John Wiley & Sons, New York

Kreitzer, Snyder (2002) Healing the heart. *Cardiovasc Nurs* **17**(2): 73–80

References

LaClave, Bix (1989) Children with cancer. *J Adolesc Healthcare* **10**: 323–27

Lelliott, *et al* (2001) *Carers and Users Expectations*. British Journal of Psychiatry, London

Ministry of Agriculture, Food and Fisheries (2000) *National Diet and Nutrition Survey*. HMSO, London

Moll A (1889) *Hypnotism*. Walter Scott, London

Morrissey M (2003) *Becoming a Mental Health Nurse*. APS Publishing, Salisbury

Needham (1893) *Report of the Committee on Hypnotism*. British Medical Journal, London

Nijhou HJ (1990) *BioEssays 1990*. John Wiley & Sons, New York: 441–46

Nolen-Hoeksema S (2001) *Abnormal Psychology*, 2nd edn. McGraw Hill, Boston

Olness, Kohen (1996) *Hypnosis and Hypnotherapy with Children*. Guildford Press, New York

Packard, Vance (1957) *The Hidden Persuaders*. David McKay & Co, Montreal

Pert *et al* (1985) *Neuropeptides and Their Receptors*. National Institute of Mental Health, London

Regal S, Roberts D (2002) *Mental Health Liaison*. Bailliere Tindall, Edinburgh

Sainsbury Centre for Mental Health (1998) Briefing Paper 4: *Acute Problems in Psychiatric Wards*. SCMH, London

Schachter (1971) Facts about human beings and rats. *Am Psychol* **26**: 129–44

Schachter, *et al* (1968) Effects of fear and food deprivation on obesity. *J Person Social Psychol* **10**: 91–97

Strathdee, *et al* (1997) A *GP's Guide to Managing Mental Health Disorders*. SCMH, London

Stuart, Sundeen, eds (1997) *Mental Health Nursing*. Butterworth Heineman, Oxford

Talbot M (2000) The Placebo Prescription. *New York Times Magazine*, January 9th

Tuckey LC (1889) *Treatment of Hypnotism and Suggestion.* Bailliere, Tindall & Cox, London

Van Wormer (2001) *Quantitative Evaluation of Hypnotically Suggested Analgesia.* Indiana School of Nursing, USA

Wakley T (1842) Mesmerism. *Lancet*: 24–13

Waterfield R (2002a) *Hidden Depths.* Macmillan, London: 75

Waterfield R (2002b) *Mesmerism in India.* Longmans, London: 199

Waterfield R (2002c) *Parodies.* Macmillan, London

Watkins P (2001) *Mental Health Nursing.* Butterworth Heineman, Oxford

World Health Organization (2001) *Guide to Mental Health in Primary Care.* Royal Society of Medicine, London

World Health Organization (2000) *Guide to Mental Health in Primary Care.* Royal Society of Medicine, London

White GM (1982) Cultural concepts of mental health. In: Marsella, White, eds. *Ethnographic Study of Cultural Knowledge of Mental Disorder.* Reidel, Dordrecht

Zahourek RP (2002) Ericksonian hypnosis in psychiatric nursing practice. *Perspect Psychiatr Care* **38**(1): 15–22

Index

Index

Index

Index

psychological studies 51
psychomotor agitation 134, 136
psychomotor retardation 135
psychoneuroimmunology 80
psychosis 75
psychosocial treatment 131
psychosomatic 52, 82
psychosomatic condition 80
psychosomatic disorder 35
psychosomatic in origin 4
psychosomatic network 53
psychotherapy
    verbally-oriented 24
psychotic disorder 127
psychotic symptoms 121, 133, 135
puberty 116

Q

quantum physics 144

R

rape 69
rapport 4
Rasputin 53
reactive depression 121
receptivity of suggestion 22
receptor/effector IMP complexes
    145
recovery 126
recurrence 126
reductionism 144
reframing 109
regression 54
relaxation 19, 92
reproduction 141
respiration 141
respiratory system
    bacteriums 143
right brain
    is imaginative, creative 52
right brain dominant 55
RNA synthesis 144
Rossi 24
Ruff 41, 53
rugby 81

S

sadness 121
sado-masochism 46
safe place
    imagery 110
sailing 81
salts 146
Sapirstein, Guy 12, 49
Schachter 114
Schmitt 24
secondary benefits 118
sedatives
    abuse of 129
self harm 108
self receptors 146
self-esteem
    inflated 136
    low 54, 68
self-healing 98
serotonin 138
sex 45
sexual assault 54
sexual drives 45
sexual response 46
sexuality
    interest in 47
shell shock 25
skiing 81
sky diving 81
sleep
    decreased need for 135
smoking 18, 56-57, 62, 77, 82
social phobia 123
Spiegel 62
splenectomy 19
spontaneous regression 63
Stanford University 11
stomach ulcers 18
stress 57, 80-81, 86, 125, 128
stroke 116, 124
Stuart 24
stutterer 39-40
subconscious 12, 43, 51-52, 54, 61,
    66, 75, 101, 108
    healing power of 83
    right brain and 52
subconscious mind 49

Printed in the United Kingdom
by Lightning Source UK Ltd.
124845UK00001B/181-222/A